THE
INSANITY
OFFENSE

ALSO BY E. FULLER TORREY

Surviving Prostate Cancer (2006)

Beasts of the Earth (2005, senior author)

Surviving Manic-Depression (2002, senior author)

The Invisible Plague: The Rise of Mental Illness from 1750 to the Present (2002, senior author)

Out of the Shadows: Confronting America's Mental Illness Crisis (1997)

Schizophrenia and Manic-Depressive Disorder (1994, senior author)

Freudian Fraud (1992)

Criminalizing the Seriously Mentally Ill (1992, senior author)

Frontier Justice: The Rise and Fall of the Loomis Gang (1992)

Nowhere to Go: The Tragic Odyssey of the Homeless Mentally Ill (1988)

Care of the Seriously Mentally Ill (1986, 1988, 1990, senior author)

Surviving Schizophrenia: A Family Manual (1983, 1988, 1995, 2001, 2006)

The Roots of Treason: Ezra Pound and the Secret of St. Elizabeths (1983)

Schizophrenia and Civilization (1980)

Why Did You Do That? (1975)

The Death of Psychiatry (1974)

Witchdoctors and Psychiatrists (1972, 1986)

Ethical Issues in Medicine (1968, editor)

THE
INSANITY
OFFENSE

How America's Failure
to Treat the
Seriously Mentally Ill
Endangers Its Citizens

E. Fuller Torrey

W. W. NORTON & COMPANY
New York • London

For information about permission to reproduce selections from this book,
write to Permissions, W. W. Norton & Company, Inc.
500 Fifth Avenue, New York, NY 10110

For information about special discounts for bulk purchases, please contact
W. W. Norton Special Sales at specialsales@wwnorton.com or 800-233-4830

Manufacturing by RR Donnelley, Bloomsburg
Book design by Dana Sloan
Production manager: Julia Druskin

Library of Congress Cataloging-in-Publication Data

Torrey, E. Fuller (Edwin Fuller), 1937–
The insanity offense : how America's failure to treat the seriously
mentally ill endangers its citizens / E. Fuller Torrey.—1st ed.
p. ; cm.
Includes bibliographical references and index.
ISBN 978-0-393-06658-6 (hardcover)
1. Mental health services—United States—Evaluation.
2. Mentally ill—Deinstitutionalization—United States.
3. Mentally ill—Commitment and detention—United States.
4. Dangerously mentally ill—United States.
5. Mental health laws—United States. I. Title.
[DNLM: 1. Commitment of Mentally Ill—United States.
2. Dangerous Behavior—United States.
3. Deinstitutionalization—United States.
4. Mental Health Services—organization & administration—United States.
5. Mentally Ill Persons—United States. WM 33 AA1 T694i 2008]
RC443.T67 2008
362.196'89—dc22

                                                            2008002697

W. W. Norton & Company, Inc.
500 Fifth Avenue, New York, N.Y. 10110
www.wwnorton.com

W. W. Norton & Company Ltd.
Castle House, 75/76 Wells Street, London W1T 3QT

1 2 3 4 5 6 7 8 9 0

For Ted and Vada Stanley,
who, through their generous support of research and
the Treatment Advocacy Center, have made a major
contribution to improving the lives of individuals with
severe psychiatric disorders.

*All royalties have been donated to the Treatment Advocacy Center and to
families who have suffered from our failure to provide treatment.*

Manifold are thy shapings, Providence!
Many a hopeless matter gods arrange.
What we expected never came to pass,
What we did not expect the gods brought to bear;
So have things gone, this whole experience through!

—*Closing chorus of Euripides'* Medea

Contents

Preface

The genesis of this book took place around 1980, when I gradually became aware that something was going terribly wrong. At the time, I was working in the public mental hospital of Washington, D.C.—St. Elizabeths—on wards with patients diagnosed with schizophrenia, bipolar disorder, major depression, and other severe psychiatric disorders. My job was to get them well, then to discharge them to the community.

I noticed that some of the patients did fine, but that many did not. The follow-up care on offer left much to be desired, and many needed frequent rehospitalizations. Some were lost to follow-up and became homeless, while others ended up in jail. A few were having their monthly disability checks stolen by the operators of their boarding homes, and one young woman I had treated was being rented out by a pimp. The death rate from suicide and neglected medical conditions among these patients seemed inordinately high.

On March 12, 1980, Dennis Sweeney shot to death former Congressman Allard Lowenstein, a charismatic leader for civil rights. Sweeney had graduated from Stanford University and worked on civil rights in the South with Lowenstein. Sweeney had then developed paranoid schizophrenia and become convinced that Lowenstein was leading an international conspiracy against him by sending voices through his dental fillings to torment him. The news clipping of this tragedy became the first entry in my "preventable tragedies" file, which was to grow over the years to fill entire file drawers. Since the year 2000, there have been almost three thousand entries.

During the 1980s and 1990s, I volunteered at a local homeless shelter and visited shelters and jails in almost half of the fifty states. Everywhere I looked, the situation was getting worse. In 1989, I learned of the killing of Malcoum Tate, who had untreated schizophrenia, by his mother and sister. I wrote to the family, offering to testify pro bono, but their lawyer declined. The enormity of the tragedy awed me, as Euripides' *Medea* had awed Athenians two and a half millennia earlier:

> *Friends, I am resolved as quickly as I can to kill the boys and leave this land: Not to delay and give them to another's hand less merciful than mine to murder. They have to die. And since they must, I who gave them birth will kill them.*

Was this to be the final measure of a failed system, the debacle that had come to be called deinstitutionalization?

I sometimes ask myself why I wrote this book, but the morning newspaper too often offers a stark reminder. On May 14, 2006, it was an account of the funeral of Vicky Armel, a forty-year-old Fairfax County, Virginia, police detective shot to death by Michael Kennedy, an eighteen-year-old with seven guns and untreated schizophrenia.[1] More than four thousand persons attended the funeral, including police officers from Pennsylvania, Ohio, and New York. Armel left behind a husband, a seven-year-old son, and a four-year-old daughter. On an inside page another headline read, "Son, 24, Charged in Mother's Death: Neighbors Say the Woman Talked about Young Man's Mental Illness." The young man, Nathan Jones, was described as "a former College of William and Mary student [who] was struggling with a mental illness that appeared to first affect him in college."[2] The murder was brutal. I knew the story without even having to read it and filed it with the hundreds of similar stories.

I have tried to convey the magnitude of this national tragedy by quantifying it. But numbers are too abstract; like the numbers of people killed by an earthquake or in a flood, they fail to communicate what it is really like for a person to be crushed to death or swept away in a deluge. Whenever possible, I have attempted to give the tragedy a human dimension.

Of all the disturbing aspects of this book, perhaps the most disturbing is the knowledge that things are worse than what I describe. I have chosen to highlight cases from California, Wisconsin, and North Carolina. In 1972 and 1973, when Herbert Mullin killed thirteen people, California was regarded as one of the leading states for mental health services. In 1986, one year after Bryan Stanley killed three people in Wisconsin, a national survey I coauthored ranked the state as one of the top three states for public psychiatric services. In 1988, when Malcoum Tate was killed by his mother and sister, North Carolina was ranked seventh in a similar national survey.[3] Instead of these states, regarded at the time as among the best, I could have chosen Texas or Louisiana, Montana or Idaho, or almost any other state where public psychiatric services are among the worst.

Ultimately, I am writing this book because I continue to hope that we can improve the outcomes for those afflicted by severe mental illnesses, for their families, and for potential victims. I am certain that if we recognize the importance of anosognosia, as described in chapter 7, and take steps to ensure that those who need treatment receive it, as outlined in chapter 11, we can markedly reduce the occurrence of tragedies like the ones described in this book. As has been said, describing a problem is the first step in solving it.

Acknowledgments

This book would not exist except for the kindness of many people. I am especially indebted to Pauline Wilkerson for sharing her family's story, despite having absolutely no reason to trust a mental health professional. Mary Stanley, Herb Mullin, and Alberta Lessard were also generous with their time and willingness to recount painful past histories.

Librarians are a writer's best friends, and Linda Johnson at the California State Archives and Janet Meyer at the Supreme Court of South Carolina were especially helpful. I am also indebted to the following for responding to my inquiries: Robert Blondis, Myron Gordon, John Justice, Matthew Large, Donald Lunde, Eugene Maloney, Hans Schanda, Greg Van Rybroek, and Thomas Zander. Various phases of the manuscript were substantially improved by critiques from Alicia Aebersold, Alec Buchanan, Faith Dickerson, Fred Frese, Carla Jacobs, Richard Lamb, Jon Stanley, Darold Treffert, and Mary Zdanowicz.

I am also grateful to Judy Miller, my research assistant, Otto Sonntag, my copyeditor, and Brendan Curry, my editor at W. W. Norton; all improved the manuscript in myriad ways through their polite but perceptive suggestions. Rafe Sagalyn, my agent, was remarkably effective. My largest debt, as always, is to Barbara Torrey, my unofficial copyeditor and wife of four decades.

In addition, I wish to thank the following:

- Laura Van Tosh, Irene Levine, and Bill MacPhee of *Schizophrenia Digest* for permission to use part of Irene Levine's article "Insight: The Key Piece in Recovery's Puzzle."
- Herschel Hardin for permission to reprint part of his essay "Uncivil Liberties," originally published in the *Vancouver Sun*.

THE

INSANITY

OFFENSE

1 | Introduction: The Origins of a Disaster

> *It must be remembered that for the person with severe mental*
> *illness who has no treatment, the most dreaded of confinements*
> *can be the imprisonment inflicted by his own mind, which shuts*
> *reality out and subjects him to the torment of voices and images*
> *beyond our powers to describe.*

SUPREME COURT JUSTICE ANTHONY KENNEDY, 1999

This book is about one of the great social disasters of recent American history. It began within the lifetime of many of us, is continuing, and today affects approximately 400,000 individuals and their families. In the annals of twentieth-century American history, it should be included among the greatest calamities.

There are two major origins of the disaster—deinstitutionalization and the legal profession. The first was a policy to move psychiatric patients out of public mental hospitals and place them in the community. This trend began following World War II, sparked by a series of exposés of dreadful conditions in state psychiatric hospitals. Massive overcrowding and a lack of effective treatments had led to conditions that were inhumane on the best of days and often much worse. Albert Maisel's 1946 pictorial exposé in *Life* magazine was followed by multiple descriptive accounts, such as Mike Gorman's *Oklahoma Attacks Its Snake Pits* and Albert Deutsch's *The Shame of the States*. The discovery

1

of effective antipsychotic drugs in the early 1950s made it possible for the first time to ameliorate the symptoms for many seriously mentally ill patients and thus to discharge them.

So began the emptying of the hospitals, first as a trickle and then as a flood, in what became known as deinstitutionalization. The emptying of psychiatric hospitals was a policy conceived by and born to parents with the best of intentions, but who then badly neglected their off-spring. Once patients were released from hospitals, essential aftercare in most places varied from inadequate to invisible.

The authors of deinstitutionalization often deny a relationship between the closing of state mental hospitals and the increase in home-lessness, incarceration, victimization, and acts of violence associated with some of the released patients. Such protestations contradict com-mon sense and ignore the obvious temporal relationship between the events. A recent study of eighty-one U.S. cities demonstrated a direct correlation between the decrease in the number of public psychiatric beds and the subsequent increase in homelessness, arrest rates, and crime rates among mentally ill individuals in those cities.[1]

It is important to understand the magnitude of deinstitutionaliza-tion. In 1955, when the United States had a population of 164 million people, there were over 558,000 mentally ill individuals in public mental hospitals. In 2006, the United States had a population of almost 300 million; if in 2006 we had had the same number of individuals in public mental hospitals as we had in 1955 in proportion to the popu-lation, the number of hospitalized patients would have been just over one million. In 2006, there were in fact only approximately 40,000 individuals in public mental hospitals. In order to understand the tragedies being described in this book, it is also necessary to appreci-ate the timing of deinstitutionalization. During the first decade, from 1956 to 1965, only 16 percent of those who would ultimately be dein-stitutionalized were released from the hospital (figure 1). Moreover, these were the patients who had the least severe symptoms and were most likely to have a supportive family and to be aware of their illness and take medication. Between 1966 and 1975, 54 percent of the patients were deinstitutionalized, and between 1976 and 1984, 18 percent more were released. Thus, three-quarters of the patients who were being deinstitutionalized left the hospitals between 1966 and 1984. The patients released in the later years tended to be those who were sicker, who had fewer social supports, and who were less likely to be aware of their illness and take medication. On the basis of this scenario, one would expect to find the earliest adverse effects of deinstitutionalization appearing in the early 1970s, then to see these effects increase sharply over the following two decades. This is exactly what we find.

Figure 1.

The Magnitude of Deinstitutionalization: Number of Patients in Public Mental Hospitals, 1950–2005

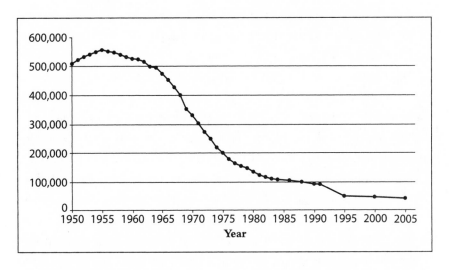

Deinstitutionalization was not a onetime experiment that might be easily reversed. Once a patient was discharged from the hospital, that bed was no longer available for that person to return to or for a new patient to use. Eventually, at least forty state mental hospitals were closed altogether. Many of the seriously mentally ill individuals described in this book who today are homeless, incarcerated, victimized, violent, or otherwise not receiving treatment have never been hospitalized at all.

The other major origin of the disaster is the legal profession. In the

1960s, at the height of the civil rights era, a small group of young lawyers focused on the fact that the civil rights of hospitalized psychiatric patients were being violated, which in many instances was true. The group included the lawyers Bruce Ennis (see chapter 5) and Thomas Zander (see chapter 6). Ennis had just completed law school and, although he had had no experience with mentally ill persons or psychiatric hospitals, decided that psychiatric hospitals were "places where sick people get sicker and sane people go mad." Ennis's avowed goal was "nothing less than the abolition of involuntary hospitalization" and the ultimate closure of all mental hospitals. In the late 1960s, Ennis and other young lawyers organized what became the Mental Health Law Project, originally under the aegis of the New York Civil Liberties Union, which passed a resolution saying that involuntary hospitalization was incompatible with the principles of a free society.[2]

Civil liberties lawyers proceeded to bring legal actions in several states targeted at closing down the hospitals. In Alabama, in *Wyatt v. Stickney*, they obtained a ruling mandating a minimum staffing ratio for treating the patients; many states achieved this ratio by simply discharging patients, not by hiring more staff. In *Donaldson v. O'Connor*, lawyers successfully sued a Florida state hospital psychiatrist on behalf of a patient they alleged had not received adequate treatment. That patient and thousands like him were discharged.

At the same time, civil liberties lawyers also brought lawsuits that sought to make it as difficult as possible to get patients back into the hospitals. In the long run, these cases were much more damaging to patient care, because they largely abolished the means to involuntarily treat individuals who would become severely mentally ill in the future. Foremost among these lawsuits was the *Lessard* decision in Wisconsin, described in chapters 5 and 6. Complementing these lawsuits were others establishing the right of psychiatric patients to refuse treatment, even if the patients did not know they were sick; representative of such suits were *Rennie v. Klein* in New Jersey and *Rogers v. Okin* in Massachusetts.

Virtually all of this legal action took place between the mid-1960s and the mid-1980s. During those same years, of course, the nation's psychiatric hospitals were being emptied. Deinstitutionalization emptied the patients from the hospitals, and the civil rights lawyers ensured that many of the patients would not be treated or rehospitalized. These two movements were like two flooding streams coming together, complementing each other and synergistically causing much more damage than either could have done alone. Downstream, the devastating effects—homelessness, incarceration, victimization, violence, and homicides—are clearly visible today.

What does this mean in terms of actual numbers? The counting of seriously mentally ill people in the United States is surprisingly imprecise. The National Mental Health Information Center estimates that 5.4 percent of people eighteen and over, or 12.8 million adults, have a "serious mental illness." The National Institute of Mental Health (NIMH) claims that 3.7 percent of people eighteen and over, or 8.8 million adults, have schizophrenia or bipolar disorder. Schizophrenia is a disease of the brain characterized most commonly by auditory hallucinations (hearing voices), delusions (e.g., thinking that people are trying to kill you), and abnormal emotions. Bipolar disorder is similar except that extreme emotions, such as mania or severe depression, are characteristic of it. An objective review of available data suggests that approximately 4 million American adults have the most severe forms of psychiatric disorders, specifically schizophrenia, bipolar disorder with psychosis, and severe depression with psychosis. This number is consistent with the fact that 3.2 million individuals were receiving federal Supplemental Security Income (SSI) or Social Security Disability Insurance (SSDI) in 2002 for "mental disorders other than mental retardation"; the vast majority of SSI and SSDI funds goes to the mentally ill individuals who are the most severely impaired.[3]

The Magnitude of the Problem

4,000,000: The number of individuals in the United States who have severe psychiatric disorders (schizophrenia, bipolar disorder with psychosis, depression with psychosis).

400,000: The subset of the 4 million that is most problematic if not treated, estimated to be approximately 10 percent of the total.

These are the individuals who are most often homeless, incarcerated, victimized, and/or violent. Most are not aware of their illness and therefore will not take medication. Most of them need to be on some form of assisted treatment.

40,000: The most overtly dangerous, 1 percent of the total. These individuals have been proven to be dangerous. They have committed violent acts and, if unmedicated, are likely to do so again. Most of them can live in the community as long as it is guaranteed that they are on medication to control their symptoms.

Among the 4 million American adults with serious psychiatric disorders is a subset of individuals who are most problematic. These are the ones who are most likely to become homeless, incarcerated, victimized, and/or violent. They include those individuals with the most severe forms of schizophrenia and bipolar disorder, and many also have problems with alcohol or drug abuse. A study of individuals with schizophrenia in England reported that the 10 percent of patients who are the most severely affected are responsible for 80 percent of the total costs for all individuals with the disease.[4] No comparable study has been undertaken in the United States. However, as will be detailed in chapter 9, the total number of seriously mentally ill individuals who at any given time are homeless (175,000) or incarcerated (218,000) is estimated to be just under 400,000, which is 10 percent of the 4 million individuals with severe psychiatric disorders. Until hard data become available, it seems reasonable to use this estimate for the subset that is most problematic.

Among this 400,000 is a subset of those who are the most dangerous. There are no studies that permit a precise statement of their number, but, on the basis of the studies detailed in chapter 9, it is reasonable to estimate that this most dangerous group includes approximately 1 percent of individuals with severe psychiatric disorders, or 40,000 individuals. These are the individuals who have previously committed homicides or other violent crimes and are currently in forensic psychiatric hospitals and prisons. They are the John Hinckleys, Andrew Goldsteins, and Russell Westons who periodically seize headlines. They should be released from hospital or prison only under conditions in which their taking of medication to control their symptoms is guaranteed. Remarkably, this is not always the case.

As will be discussed in chapter 11, it is possible to identify the approximately 400,000 most problematic and 40,000 most dangerous individuals with severe psychiatric disorders. Geographically, they are not distributed equally but tend to be concentrated in large cities and in neighborhoods in which large numbers of discharged patients live. Such numbers are hopeful insofar as they quantify the problem. Every state mental health authority can realistically identify and provide treatment for these most problematic and dangerous individuals. The deinstitutionalization disaster of the last four decades can be reversed. There is no question that we have the means and ability to do so. The question, rather, is whether we have the will.

"People Will . . . Be Shocked and Appalled"

On January 3, 1999, a pleasant Sunday afternoon in New York City, Andrew Goldstein became one of the most highly publicized failures of the American psychiatric care system. Goldstein pushed Kendra Webdale, a young woman he had never met, to her death under the wheels of an oncoming subway train. Goldstein had a ten-year history of schizophrenia with a 3,500-page psychiatric record. According to this record, "he had been hospitalized 13 times after making unprovoked attacks on 13 individuals," including a woman and a child in a bookstore, two strangers in a Burger King, a nurse, a doctor, and a woman in a subway car. His clinical records labeled him a "high risk for violence." While hospitalized, he responded well to antipsychotic medication but rarely took it unless he was supervised and made to do so. He had been discharged from a hospital just three weeks before the murder. Over the years, he had received at least $65,000 in disability checks, and his multiple short-term hospitalizations in 1998 alone had cost $95,075 in public (mostly Medicaid) funds. Goldstein, however, was never required to continue taking the medication that kept him from being violent. At one of Goldstein's court hearings, a judge said, "I have no doubt that someday . . . people will look at our treatment of mental illness and be shocked and appalled."

> *M. Winerip: "Long before Andrew Goldstein pushed a woman in front of a train, he pleaded for help; he couldn't get it,"* New York Times Magazine, *May 23, 1999; "Oddity and normality vie in killer's taped confession,"* New York Times, *October 18, 1999; "Man who pushed woman onto tracks needed supervision, report says," ibid., November 5, 1999.*

2 | Death by the Roadside

*The paramount civil right of the patient should be
that of adequate treatment.*

STEPHEN RACHLIN, 1974

Among her nine, Malcoum Tate was Pauline Wilkerson's best child.[1]
According to her, "he was different from all the others because he
never told stories, he always told the truth. I knew he was different from
the beginning." In the Baltimore schools, he got good grades and his teachers said he was one of the smartest. One teacher told Ms. Wilkerson that
she didn't even have to bother coming to the parent-teacher conferences,
because Malcoum was doing so well.

In fact, it was hard for Pauline Wilkerson to attend school meetings.
Since her ex-husbands did not provide much help, she was often working two jobs as a domestic in order to support her family. She was a
determined but practical woman whose life skills had been honed by
sixty-one challenging years. She didn't drink, smoke, or use drugs and
had devoted her life to providing for her children. She was fiercely
devoted to members of her family and would do anything to protect
them. As she later sadly phrased it, "Sometimes you just do what you
have to do."

When he was growing up, Malcoum had gotten along well with his
brothers and sisters. His sister Lothell, three years younger, idolized her

big brother. That all changed when, in 1970, Malcoum turned sixteen and God started talking to him. Initially, this did not cause problems, except that he dropped out of school and began to drink and occasionally to smoke marijuana. His brothers tried to look out for him. One brother recalled, "I was embarrassed by him because everyone knew he was the crazy dude."[2]

As he grew older, Malcoum began receiving more specific instructions from God. Malcoum had a mission, he claimed, and if he didn't carry it out many innocent people might die. On one occasion, Malcoum was in the car with his mother when they stopped at Wilson Street for a red light. Malcoum looked around and saw the name Wilson on a mailbox. He started thinking that this was too strange to be a mere coincidence, that something odd was going on in the house, so he jumped out of the car and broke into the house and began beating a man who had been reading in a chair. Malcoum later claimed that he thought the man was the brother of [Ugandan] President Idi Amin. This 1977 episode led to Malcoum's first psychiatric hospitalization. At Maryland's Springfield State Hospital, he was described in the hospital records as being intermittently mute, hallucinating, incoherent, and offering a "confusing and rambling account" of his behavior. He was diagnosed with acute schizophrenia and deemed "dangerous." He remained involuntarily hospitalized for five months, during which time he was treated with antipsychotic medications that produced a marked improvement in his condition.

After being discharged, Malcoum returned to Baltimore to live with his mother. Although given appointments for follow-up care at the North Baltimore Mental Health Center and strongly urged to continue taking his medication, he refused to do so. He said he didn't trust the people in the clinic, and he thought the medication would kill him. The messages from God soon returned, and he became convinced that he was Malcolm X. He felt that he was blessed by God, so he started preaching to people in the street, telling them about the judgment of God and the meanings of the Koran.

Within several months, Malcoum's behavior deteriorated. He was charged with disorderly conduct for acting bizarrely on the roof of a building, and readmitted to Springfield State Hospital for another five months. He was diagnosed with chronic schizophrenia and said to be "grossly paranoid and excessively preoccupied with religious themes."

After his second hospital discharge, Malcoum again declined to take medication or participate in any follow-up care. He was six feet, two inches tall, strong, and determined to refuse treatment. At the time, Maryland was, and to this day continues to be, one of the few states with no law allowing for outpatient commitment. Under these laws, individuals like Malcoum can be legally required to take medication to control their psychiatric symptoms; if they fail to do so, they can be involuntarily rehospitalized. Ms. Wilkerson made endless inquiries regarding how to get psychiatric help for Malcoum, only to be told that nothing could be done until he demonstrated that he was dangerous. The Wilson Street incident did not qualify as "dangerous" in Maryland, because it was no longer considered a recent event.

Despairing of getting help for Malcoum in Maryland, Pauline Wilkerson in 1982 moved her family to Gastonia, North Carolina, where she had worked as a young woman. Gastonia was just across the state line from Clover, South Carolina, where she had grown up and where her mother, father, and sister were living. Malcoum was twenty-eight years old at the time of the move and appeared to be getting sicker. Previously, he had talked about seeing people on the bus, like movie stars and singers, and preached to people on the street. Now he began increasingly to focus on his mission.

Malcoum explained his mission as follows: "I am a prophet from God. God done sent me here and I have got to rid the world of all these evil people." He accused his entire family of being evil but especially focused on his niece N'Zinga, Lothell's daughter. Repeatedly, Malcoum had said, "N'Zinga is the first one I am going to rid the world of. N'Zinga is the devil, she got Satan in her and He [God] has done sent me down here to kill her." On one occasion, Malcoum took N'Zinga and disappeared for several hours. Lothell was terrified until N'Zinga was returned unharmed, but she could not forget what had happened. N'Zinga was the most important thing in her life, a life marked by intermittent drug use and severe, insulin-dependent diabetes. Lothell's doctor had told her she probably would not live to be forty; he would be right. Lothell later recalled,

> *All he [Malcoum] talked about was ridding people—ridding the world of evil people and we were all Satan and he was God and I was scared. I was scared for my daughter, because he constantly talked about her all the time, he talked about how evil she was and he talked about my mother, he talked about how no good she was and that he was going to have to do something. . . . He would walk around and he would talk to himself and I would hear him say things to himself like "something has got to be done, something has got to be done."*[3]

Over the next two years, Malcoum Tate became progressively more agitated and threatening. By 1984, he was being arrested regularly for a variety of offenses, mostly related to his worsening symptoms. During one five-month period, he was arrested and jailed seven separate times for threatening behavior, public intoxication, disturbing the peace, trespassing, breaking and entering, and larceny (stealing a 35-cent pack of crackers). As Lothell later recalled, "every three or four days they were locking him up for something." He was regularly referred to the local mental health center, where he was seen about twenty times. He was given medication, which he would take for a few days and show improvement. Invariably, he would stop taking it, according to the center's director, because he didn't perceive himself as being sick, and therefore became psychotic again.

On two occasions in 1984, Malcoum was involuntarily hospitalized at North Carolina's Broughton State Hospital. On the first occasion, he was picked up by the police for walking in the middle of a highway, oblivious of the traffic. According to the hospital records, he told the police that "he trusted Allah that he would not get hurt." The police took him to the emergency room, where he came in "laughing and singing, and then suddenly went berserk. He tried to choke a security guard and threw chairs and tables everywhere" because "the T.V. was giving special messages to him." He had to be "restrained, handcuffed and tied up" in order to be transported to the state hospital fifty miles away. Five days later, Malcoum was discharged from the hospital and said to be no longer dangerous. The psychiatrist had prescribed antipsychotic medication, and Malcoum refused to take it, so the psychiatrist discharged him.

One month later, Malcoum was involuntarily readmitted to Broughton, again said to be a danger to himself and others. The hospital notes indicate that he "admitted to threatening his mother" and that he was preoccupied with "demon possession." This time, he was treated with 100 mg of chlorpromazine, an inadequate dose for most patients with severe schizophrenia, and released after ten days. The hospital's treatment philosophy was reflected by a public comment made by its director: "It comes down to a philosophical view: Do people have a right to be crazy?"[4]

A Cry for Help, Unheard

In December 1984, Pauline Wilkerson's view of the danger her son posed was permanently altered. The Gastonia area media heavily publicized the brutal murder of Emily Cannon, a Charlotte high school history teacher, by her son who had schizophrenia. Bobby Cannon had been a Boy Scout and model student who was "well-dressed, quiet and polite,"[5] the only child in what neighbors described as a perfect family in which "he and his mother would always go bicycle riding together."

In his senior year in high school, Bobby Cannon developed schizophrenia and became violent. He called his mother names and told friends that she was "messing with my mind." Shortly after the onset of his illness, he attacked his mother and threatened to kill her with a screwdriver. He was hospitalized but discharged after one week. A week later, he beat both his mother and father with a board; his mother was hospitalized for a week with head injuries, and his father was treated for lacerations. Bobby Cannon was again hospitalized and then released.

For the next two years, the Cannons did everything possible to get psychiatric help for their son. He said he was God, refused treatment, and became periodically violent. He was jailed and finally given anti-psychotic medication that produced substantial improvement. In September 1984, however, a psychiatrist at the mental health center discontinued his medication, erroneously concluding that Cannon did not have schizophrenia but rather that his symptoms had been induced by street drugs.

On December 1, Emily Cannon addressed a letter to nine mental health officials and county commissioners, pleading for help for her son. She recounted the family's multiple failed efforts to get help for him. Ever since his medication had been discontinued, she wrote, "he insisted on having an axe in his room while he slept," and he had "started looking for a bat and said he was going to kill the first person in sight." Ms. Cannon concluded her letter to the public officials,

> *Please remember that one of the most important things that can be done now and in the future is to make sure that those hired to work with the mentally ill are sensitive and caring human beings. Sensitive to the needs of patients, families, this country, this state and mankind.*

Four days after Emily Cannon wrote the letter, her son beat her to death with a vacuum cleaner. He then slashed her body with a butcher knife and dumped it in woods north of Charlotte. When he was arrested, police reported that Bobby claimed "he was told by God that he had to kill his mother and he does not seem to see anything wrong with what he did because it was ordered by God."

Pauline Wilkerson vividly recalled hearing about the Cannon case. "That sounds like my son," she had said. "I had a feeling it was coming—he was going to kill us all." She was haunted by what Bobby Cannon had done, and she knew that if a schoolteacher like Emily Cannon had not been able to get help her chances were even worse. Lothell Tate later recalled, "That's all she would talk about, how that woman, knowing the people that she knows, she couldn't get no help for that boy, and here she is, somebody that's a domestic worker, and she keeps asking, keeps asking, and nobody does anything."[6]

* * *

The three years following the murder of Emily Cannon were increasingly terrifying for Pauline Wilkerson and her family. Malcoum was convinced that he was God and had a divine mission to rid the world of all evil. He told his family that he was making a plan and was going to take care of it. He wandered through the house during the night, and family members often awoke to find Malcoum standing over them. Lothell recalled, "I woke up one night and he was standing up over my bed, just smiling, and I said, 'Malcoum, what are you doing?' and he just looked at me and smiled and walked out of the room. . . . This would happen two or three times out of the week." Pauline Wilkerson also experienced this "too many times to count," awakening in the middle of the night with her son standing over her. "He would give a strange laugh and then walk away." It terrified her, and she began to sleep at friends' homes whenever she could.

Malcoum's behavior also became less predictable. He sometimes put things on the stove and forgot about them. On one morning, he set fire to the kitchen. N'Zinga spotted the flames and woke everyone up; they got out safely, but the kitchen was badly damaged. Malcoum's aggressive behavior and threats were also increasing. He "started calling his mother a bitch and a slut. Some days he'd call her at work just to tell her that."[7] His threats to kill N'Zinga and the rest of the family escalated to a virtual daily occurrence. According to his mother, he often said, "Mama, you just remember now that when I'm killing you, it's not really me who is doing it but God."

During these months, Pauline Wilkerson tried endlessly to get help for her son. According to Lothell,

> *My mother would get on the phone and she would call all of these agencies, these help organizations that are there to help people, and every time she would call and talk to them, they would say, "Oh, let him take his medication; he will be all right." She would say, "Well, he is not taking his medication," and they would say, "Well, you are going to have to make him take his medication, Ms. Wilkerson."*

But there was no way to make Malcoum take his medication, since he believed he was God. His mother, sisters, and brothers pleaded with him to take it. Occasionally he would, for a few days, but usually he simply replied, "Hell, no, I won't take it. I don't need no medicine."

Calls to the local mental health center were equally futile. Responses were always variations on the same theme: they said there was nothing they could do with Malcoum until he became violent. Pleas to the personnel at Broughton State Hospital to keep Malcoum long enough to get him stabilized on medication merely elicited the response that they had guidelines, and if Malcoum was not violent and hadn't done anything to hurt anybody, they couldn't keep him. The "guidelines" referred to were "clear, cogent and convincing evidence" of being a danger to yourself or others. It was always the same—"until," "until," "until"—it was this constant "until" that Pauline Wilkerson and her family found terrifying.

In 1987, Malcoum Tate returned to Baltimore, where he had grown up. He had saved $1,500 from his SSI disability checks and had decided that he could better accomplish God's mission in his old neighborhood. For his family, it was to be but a brief respite. A few days after his arrival in the city, according to Lothell, "he called back and said he didn't have any money and he had left the door open to the apartment and that some people had come in and stole everything that he had and that he had started drinking." His sister asked, "Malcoum, have you been taking your medication?" and he replied, "No, I am not taking medication no more, Lothell, because I don't need no medication. All I need is God and my wine bottle."

Two days later, Malcoum was in the Baltimore County Jail. According to Lothell, he had been arrested because "he was on an elevator with a Caucasian lady and he wanted to know what time it was, so he grabbed the lady's arm to see what time it was and she started screaming and yelling and said he attacked her and they threw him in jail for that." Lothell went to Baltimore to explain to the police that Malcoum was sick and shouldn't be prosecuted as a criminal; he was therefore released and advised to seek psychiatric treatment.

After Malcoum returned to Gastonia, his condition worsened.

"He'd take showers five times a day with his clothes on" and said aliens were talking to him: "He said it was space people talking to him to populate and breed—get women. Like they had give him some kind of operation and he was going to make a new strain of life."[8]

He also became increasingly violent. While wandering the streets, according to court records, "he would disturb people . . . he would agitate them so to the point they would start fighting him and beating him up and he would come home bloody, beat up . . ." One police report noted that Malcoum had "disrupted the entire neighborhood, trespassed on property after being forbidden to do so, threatened to kill everybody."

At home, Lothell testified, "he was very vulgar in his mouth; he would cuss you out; he would throw things at you and this was very disturbing to us because we never seen him like this, never. . . . I had never seen him like this in all the years that he had been sick. We could always tell, we could always know what was going to happen, but this time it was different." Garnell Wilkerson, Malcoum's younger brother, who was away at college, also recalled his becoming "more and more violent each time I came home. I could see a change in him, and he would be more angry, and more hostile toward everyone in the family. . . . Every other sentence he would say something referring to God and getting rid of all of us."[9] Day after day, Malcoum reminded his family of his mission, to rid the world of evil people. And they were to be the first.

In late November 1988, events appeared to be moving toward some unknown dénouement. As Lothell recounted,

One night there was just me and my daughter home and it was about two or three o'clock in the morning and I was half asleep and half awake because I thought I heard somebody banging on the door, banging on the door, and by the time I got myself together to realize it was somebody banging on the door, Malcoum took his foot and kicked the door off the hinges and when I came downstairs, I said, "Malcoum, why did you do that?" He said "Well, you all should have opened the door and let me in; you all heard me banging on the door. You can't keep me out; I told you I am God; you can't do nothing to me." By this time he had made so much confusion in the apartment that . . . someone else called the police and they came and they took Malcoum to jail. Malcoum looked at me and said, "Ain't nothing going to be done to me; they can't nothing be done to me," and they took him away. So we went back to bed, my daughter was crying, she was upset, she was scared he was coming back because she was scared of him by this time. The phone rung and it was Malcoum on the other end and he was laughing and he said, "See I told you; I am out of jail; you can't do nothing to me; you can't do nothing to me; I am coming back; I am out." And that whole night I didn't sleep because I was scared. I could not believe that he was out after kicking the door down and that's a violent act, to me that is a violent act. So that morning I didn't sleep; I didn't go to work.

This episode was too much for the management of the Greenview Meadows Apartments, the two-story townhouses where Pauline Wilkerson and her family were living. When Malcoum had removed the bulbs from the outside lights of the apartments because God told him to save electricity, the management had been understanding. But kicking down doors in the middle of the night was too much, so Pauline Wilkerson and her family were given a notice of eviction. By itself, it was not the cause, merely a final straw that led Malcoum's mother and sister to a desperate act of self-preservation.

After Malcoum had broken down the door and been released by the police, Pauline Wilkerson went once again to the county mental health office to seek help. This time they agreed that he needed hospitalization. During this, his third hospitalization at Broughton, doctors noted that he was "out of touch with reality, hallucinating, and hearing God telling him to kill everybody." He was also described as having "paranoid grandiose delusions," disorganized thought processes, and grossly inappropriate emotions. He exhibited, in short, the classic symptoms of severe, untreated paranoid schizophrenia. He was restarted on antipsychotics and discharged eight days later with an admonition to take his medications and avoid alcohol.

Members of his family were deeply disappointed to see him discharged so quickly, especially since they believed that he had exhibited overtly violent behavior. As Lothell recalled, the family had hoped he would be there "for ninety days or sixty days, at least, so the medication could get in his system and start working." Even while hospitalized, according to Lothell,

> *he called home; he threatened people; he talked about how no good we were, why we put him in there, there ain't nothing wrong with him and he's going to get out of there. And sure enough after eight days, Malcoum was out and they had given him three more medications to go with the two he was already [supposed to be] taking. This was a combination of five medications they wanted him to take and he didn't have no supervision, nobody to tell him when to take it, how to take it, and he wasn't taking anything. He was drinking alcohol, ripping and running and terrorizing me and my daughter and my mother.*

After his discharge from the hospital on November 23, 1988, Malcoum was arrested "two or three times." On the last occasion, according to Lothell,

> *He called me on the telephone one night about eleven o'clock and he was crying on the phone and he said, "Lothell, you have got to get me out of here." He said, "People in here are doing things to me and I don't want to be in here; you have got to get me out of here." And I lay there and I just thought about him being in that cell by himself being sick and then when my mother came home, I said, "Mama, go get Malcoum out of jail because he said people are down there doing things to him and he don't want to be in there." So she went and got him out and he promised that he was going to stop drinking; he promised that he was going to take his medication, but as soon as he got out, and we said, "Malcoum, you said you were going to take your medication." He said a cuss word and he said, "I ain't taking nothing; I am going to get me a bottle of wine" and he went and got some wine and he got to drinking and throwing things around the house.*

The family was out of options. It was being evicted from yet another apartment because of Malcoum's behavior, and it seemed likely that he would kick the door down and follow his relatives wherever they moved. Malcoum's aunt, with whom he had sometimes stayed, had obtained a court order prohibiting him from coming to her home. He had been jailed countless times but had received no treatment and had probably been sexually abused. His family had talked with him, pleaded with him, more times than anyone could remember. As Lothell later summarized it,

> *I can't think of nothing else we could have done. We tried moving; we tried asking people for help; we tried to talk to him ourselves; I tried to talk to him. I would sit him down because we always had a good relationship, me and Malcoum, and I tried to talk to him. I tried to tell him what he was doing. I tried to say that he was hurting me, that he was hurting my mother and all of our family, and he would sit there and listen like he understood what I was saying, but he would get right up and do the same thing. No, I don't think—I tried everything. I tried to do different things, but I didn't know anything else to do. I didn't know anything else to do and I did not want nothing to happen to my daughter and he seemed too bent on how much she had the devil in her.*

"It Is Over Now"

It was difficult to remember who had initially suggested it, since it had been on both their minds. They had discussed it intermittently, obliquely, reluctantly, for several weeks. The idea would be verbalized, rejected for a day or two, then return. By mid-December 1988, it had become a question no longer of if, merely when.

On Saturday, one week before Christmas, Malcoum asked to return to Baltimore. Pauline Wilkerson and Lothell were busy moving but told him that if he returned later in the evening, they would drive him there. Malcoum returned at 11 p.m., wearing several shirts and pairs of pants. Despite the extra clothing, his strength was apparent, the product of almost daily weight lifting. He had used some of his SSI disability money to buy a membership in a health club, where he worked out but

frightened other members with his bizarre behavior. The manager of
the club would later say that he was afraid to ever turn his back on Malcoum. When Malcoum arrived that evening, he smelled of Wild Irish
Rose, his favorite drink, but he appeared less agitated than usual.

Pauline climbed into the driver's seat of their old Datsun, Malcoum
claimed the passenger seat, and Lothell sat in the back. The apartments
of Greenview Meadows sported festive window decorations in prepa-
ration for Christmas. Lothell fingered the .25-caliber revolver in her
purse. She and her mother had bought it two weeks earlier at Kent's
Pawn Shop, at the corner of Franklin and Marietta. Neither woman
had handled a gun before, so the man had showed them how to load it
and put the safety clip on. A left onto Rolling Meadows, a right on
Efird, a left on Marietta, then a quick right over the tracks on Clyde,
and they were on South York Road, Route 321.

Quiknit Crafting Inc., at the corner of Clyde and South York, represents Gastonia's glorious past. It is a remnant of the county's 104
textile mills in the 1940s, when Gaston County was economically pros-
perous. By 1988, Gastonia's jobs had gone to Mexico and Southeast
Asia, and most of the mills were empty husks. A water tower at the
edge of town advertised Gastonia as an "All American City," which it
was, as a representative of the Rust Belt. Even the water tower was
rusty.

Gastonia lies seven miles north of the South Carolina state line.
Pauline drove south on Route 321. According to Lothell's later testimony, Malcoum was talking as usual, "saying crazy things like he always
say . . . it was out of his head things he was saying." Pauline occasionally replied, while Lothell sat silently in back. They passed the Mighty
Dollar, the American Coin Laundry, the usual assortment of fast-food
restaurants, and the Calvary Baptist Church, which advertised itself as
"A Place to Begin Anew."

Four miles south of the state line, Route 321 passes through Clover,
Pauline's hometown. She had been born on a farm nearby, one of
eleven children. Her grandfather had been a slave on a local farm, and
her father had grown cotton and sugarcane to feed the family. She had
graduated from Clover High School and soon thereafter had become

pregnant with her first child. She stopped the car in York, nine miles farther south, to buy Malcoum some candy and a soda. It was almost midnight.

A mile past York, Pauline turned right on State Route 49 and they soon entered a sparsely populated area in which scrub pine and kudzu fight for supremacy. Pauline knew the stretch well, having regularly visited a friend who lived nearby in recent years. Six miles west, the road passes through Sharon, then eight miles farther comes to State Route 97. The Datsun was going so slowly that a state policeman pulled them over and asked what the trouble was. Pauline told him that she was just tired, and he let her go with a polite warning.

Route 97 passes from York to Chester County just south of Route 49, then goes over Turkey Creek and Susybole Creek. There are almost no houses in this area, and those that exist are dark in the middle of the night. This is where Malcoum announced that he needed to stop to relieve himself. Pauline pulled to the side at the top of a slight rise, just past Susybole Creek. The night was partly cloudy, with a first-quarter moon; the temperature was in the thirties.

Malcoum got out and walked toward the shoulder, which sloped downward toward a shallow ravine. He did not hear Lothell come up behind him. As she later recounted, she said, "'Malcoum, I love you and I only want the best for you and I am sorry,' and I shot him and I shot him again." Malcoum cried, "Whatcha doing, whatcha doing?" and took several steps back toward the car. Lothell shot four more times, and Malcoum fell.

She continued, "I thought if I had just shot him a couple of times that he would have died and it would have been over with, but he didn't die, he just kept moving; and I didn't want him to lay there and suffer. . . . I wasn't doing it to hurt him and I loved him and I was trying to take him out of his misery." So Lothell reloaded the gun, "and I turned my head and I just shot the gun." The autopsy would show thirteen bullet wounds—five in the back, three in the right arm, one in the left hand, three beneath the scalp, and one in the brain. After that, Lothell said, "I did bend down and I felt to see if he was still living and I said, 'May God have mercy on your soul,' and I was crying."

Lothell and her mother rolled Malcoum's body down the slope to the bottom of the ravine. They covered it with leaves and an empty dog food bag that they found there. Lothell recalled, "I was crying and . . . my mother said, 'Come on. It is over now; he is better off where he is now,' and we got into the car" and drove back to Gastonia.

3 | Thirteen Murders to Prevent an Earthquake

> *Civil libertarians say no—that it is our right to commit crimes*
> *that land us in prison, that it is our choice to be so ill that we*
> *prefer to forage through garbage and live on the streets, that it is*
> *our prerogative to let voices in our heads torment us into sleepless*
> *nights. But something tells me that the people locked up in San*
> *Quentin with a mental illness, and the people roving the back*
> *alleys of skid row, are not singing "God Bless America."*

JIM RANDALL, 2006

I t was a strange week, even by the singular standards of Santa Cruz. Regular customers at Noah's New York Bagels on Pacific Avenue speculated; other residents stayed home, even avoiding friends with whom they regularly socialized. One didn't know whom to trust anymore.

On Monday, February 12, 1973, the "skeletal remains" of a Cabrillo College student were found; the *Santa Cruz Sentinel* noted that it was "the eighth [body] found in Santa Cruz County in the last two months." On Tuesday, seventy-two-year-old Fred Perez was shot to death while working in his yard. A Marine veteran of World War I, Perez belonged to one of the town's oldest families and was known and liked by many in the community. The *Sentinel* headlined, "Senseless Slaying of Santa Cruz Man."[1]

By Wednesday, everyone knew that twenty-five-year-old Herb

Mullin had been arrested for the Perez killing. Mullin was one of their own. He had graduated in 1965 from the local high school, 27th in a class of 277, played football, basketball, and baseball, served as vice president of the Varsity Club, and been a member of the honorary Key Club. He had worked at Vic and Bill's Service Station and Johnnie's Supermarket and had gone steady with Loretta Ricketts. According to the *Sentinel*, he had been "extremely popular going through school," "a real nice kid, really bright and deeply religious."[2] The only trouble he had had in high school was the time he got caught with beer in his car.

On Thursday, Mullin was charged with five more murders. Three weeks earlier, Jim and Joan Gianera had been shot and stabbed to death in their home, the latter as she was emerging from the shower. A few miles away from the Gianera home, Kathy Francis and her two young sons had been shot and stabbed to death in their home. There had been speculation that the murders were drug-related, since more than a few Santa Cruz residents were into drugs.

On Friday, Mullin was tied to the murder of Father Henri Tomei, a Catholic priest. Father Tomei had been active in the French underground in World War II and came to California late in life. Three months earlier, he had been brutally stabbed in the confessional of Saint Mary's Catholic Church in nearby Los Gatos. Authorities found Herb Mullin's fingerprints on the confessional.

Four more bodies were found over the weekend, and Herb Mullin was charged with the murders. Nineteen-year-old Scott Card, along with Rob Spector and Dave Oliker, both eighteen, and Mark Dreibelbis, fifteen, had been camping at a remote site in the state park near Mullin's home. All had been shot to death the previous week, but their bodies were not found until Scott's brother had gone looking for them.

On Tuesday, February 20, the county district attorney, Peter Chang, was quoted in the *Sentinel* labeling Santa Cruz, a town of 32,000 persons, "the murder capital of the world."[3] Mullin was charged with eleven murders. Within two weeks, the number would swell to thirteen. One was Mary Guilfoyle, the Cabrillo College student whose remains had been found on February 12. Mullin had picked her up hitchhiking and stabbed her to death. The other victim was Lawrence

White, a drifter who had been bludgeoned to death with a baseball bat the previous October. White had been Mullin's first victim.

It wasn't supposed to be that way, especially not in Santa Cruz. The "longhairs," as they were often referred to by older residents, had taken over in the early 1960s, and peace symbols dominated the town. The students at the University of California at Santa Cruz were known as the most liberal in the state, and members of the city council were reputed to smoke marijuana during their deliberations. Isolated from the rest of California by the Santa Cruz Mountains, the town was imbued with an atmosphere of live and let live. The Elysian forests overlooking the Pacific Ocean were not supposed to spawn a "homicidal maniac," as District Attorney Chang publicly called Mullin.[4]

Herb Mullin's transition from "a real nice kid, really bright and deeply religious" in 1965 to a "homicidal maniac" responsible for thirteen murders in 1973 had been gradual. Friends noticed some changes during his second year at Cabrillo College, where he was pursuing an engineering degree. Mullin, a devout Catholic, became increasingly obsessed with Eastern religions and especially reincarnation. Over the next several months, he dropped out of college and began using marijuana more heavily. On one occasion he was arrested for possession. He tried LSD and began spending time with peers he had previously ridiculed.

There were other changes as well. In the past, Herb had expressed plans to use his engineering skills to join the Army Corps of Engineers, but instead he applied for conscientious-objector status and joined demonstrations against the war in Vietnam. For his father, who had fought proudly in World War II, this change was especially incomprehensible. During these months, Herb also broke his engagement to his longstanding girlfriend, Loretta Ricketts, and had a homosexual encounter. Mullin's family and friends saw that he was drifting, that something was wrong, but *what* was wrong remained unclear.

The answer came in the spring of 1969, shortly before Mullin's twenty-second birthday. While visiting his sister in Sonoma County, north of San Francisco, he propositioned both her and her husband. He also expressed a belief that his sister was communicating with him by telepathy. During one dinner, Herb mimicked his brother-in-law's every movement, a behavior clinicians call echopraxia. It was by then clear that something was profoundly wrong, and Herb's sister persuaded him to voluntarily admit himself to Mendocino State Hospital. There, his diagnosis was given as schizophrenia, possibly exacerbated by drug use.

Herb Mullin remained at the hospital for six weeks. He acknowledged hearing voices that sometimes told him to do things and referred to these orders as "cosmic emanations." He was treated with chlorpromazine (Thorazine) and trifluoperazine (Stelazine), standard pharmacological treatment for schizophrenia at that time, and the drugs apparently produced some improvement. He was said, however, to have been "generally uncooperative with the treatment program at Mendocino,"[5] and on May 9, 1969, he was discharged at his own request. In his report on Mullin, the discharging psychiatrist wrote, "prognosis is poor."

Mullin drifted between jobs for the next six months before again being hospitalized. He drove to San Luis Obispo to visit a friend, who became alarmed by Herb's condition. Mullin said he heard voices commanding him to do things, including shaving his head and burning his penis, which he dutifully did with a cigarette lighter. Herb also made homosexual advances to his friend. Alarmed by Herb's behavior, the friend called his physician uncle, and on October 31, Halloween, they had Herb psychiatrically examined and subsequently committed to the San Luis Obispo General Hospital psychiatric ward, where he was said to be "a danger to others, a danger to himself and gravely disabled." Since he was involuntarily committed, in contrast to the situation in Mendocino, he could not sign himself out of the hospital. He was again treated with Thorazine and Stelazine. Despite having a prognosis termed "grave" and clearly being a very sick young man, Mullin was discharged after only twenty-three days. The main reason for his dis-

charge was a law that had recently been passed by the California legislature and that was destined to become a symbol for the failure of
deinstitutionalization.

The Lanterman-Petris-Short Act

Herb Mullin's psychiatric hospitalizations could not have come at a less
opportune time for receiving the long-term treatment he needed. On
July 1, 1969, between his hospitalizations at Mendocino and San Luis
Obispo, the California Community Mental Health Services Act took
effect. It was widely known as the Lanterman-Petris-Short Act, after
the names of its sponsors in the legislature, and many abbreviated it
simply to LPS. According to one assessment, LPS brought about "the
broadest changes in the procedures for the involuntary commitment of
the mentally disordered since the process began in the early 1800s."
The law restricted involuntary psychiatric hospitalizations to a maximum of seventeen days unless the individual could be shown to be
"imminently dangerous," in which case hospitalizations could be
extended for ninety additional days. The criteria for such extended
hospitalizations were very strict; as one of its sponsors explained, "physical evidence of danger must be displayed in a court of law."[6]

Herb Mullin, although overtly and severely ill, did not meet the
new criteria for extended involuntary hospitalization under LPS. He
was receiving telepathic messages and command hallucinations, and he
was behaving strangely by propositioning his sister, brother-in-law, and
a close friend, but there was no evidence of the "imminent dangerousness" needed to keep and treat him for more than seventeen days.
Under the previous California law, Mullin could have been kept in the
hospital and treated for being "of such mental condition . . . [as being]
in need of supervision, treatment, care or restraint." That more liberal
criterion was no longer operant, however, as the sponsors of the new
commitment law had clearly intended.

The Lanterman-Petris-Short Act, which limited the treatment
options for individuals like Herb Mullin, was the product of a pro-

foundly unholy alliance. On one side was Frank Lanterman, a power-ful Republican assemblyman who called himself "a conservative cur-mudgeon."[7] For many years, he had represented Pasadena, the heartland of California's anti–mental health movement. This movement had first surfaced in 1953 when Ms. Gene Birkeland, a Los Angeles leader of a conservative group called Minute Women, U.S.A., began publicly com-paring American psychiatric hospitals to Russian concentration camps. The hospitals, she claimed, were used to keep American "political pris-oners under the guise of care and treatment of mental cases." She tes-tified before the California legislature and a U.S. Senate subcommittee. Her cry of "Siberia, U.S.A." became the slogan for other conservative groups opposed to psychiatry.

In Southern California, these groups included the Daughters of the American Revolution (DAR) and the John Birch Society. DAR branded mental health treatment "a Marxist weapon" and alleged that 80 percent of American psychiatrists were foreigners, "most of them educated in Russia." The John Birch Society also distributed literature claiming that "mental health programs are part of a Communist plot to control the people's minds," and in 1958 it erected a large billboard in Los Angeles with the following message:

> It is amazing and appalling how many supposedly intelligent people have been duped by such COMMUNIST SCHEMES AS FLUORIDA-TION and "Mental Health," especially since both the AMERICAN LEGION and the D.A.R. have publicly branded "Mental Health" as a COMMUNIST PLOT to take over our country.[8]

A distrust of psychiatry, and especially of involuntary commitment to psychiatric hospitals, thus came naturally to Frank Lanterman. It was part of the politically conservative culture of Southern California that would influence Richard Nixon and Ronald Reagan as well. Down-sizing California's state mental hospitals also had a fiscal appeal to con-servative politicians, since the mental health sector was a large and growing item in the state budget, providing care in 1955 for over 37,000 individuals. In 1965, the U.S. Congress had created Medicaid

and Medicare, which provided benefits for mentally disabled individuals who were living in the community. Persons in state psychiatric hospitals, however, were not eligible for these benefits. By discharging
patients from state hospitals and putting them in community settings,
states could effectively shift much of the cost of their care from the state
to the federal government. It did not take long for conservative state
legislators to exploit the fiscal advantages inherent in restricting admissions to state psychiatric hospitals.

At the time the Lanterman-Petris-Short Act was under consideration, many conservative politicians distrusted psychiatry on the basis of
a belief that "mental health practitioners encourage immorality, sin, and
social disorganization."[9] This was the late 1960s, and San Francisco's
Haight-Ashbury was in full psychedelic swing. Ken Kesey was promoting drug use among California's youth; Paul Goodman was promoting
anarchism in the name of mental health on Berkeley's campus; and
mental health practitioners were promoting nudity and sexual experi-
mentation at Esalen, in Big Sur. To conservatives, it appeared that Sodom
had been reborn in northern California with mental health professionals acting as midwives.

The other half of the alliance behind the Lanterman-Petris-Short
Act was led by Nicholas Petris, an ultra-liberal Democrat from Oakland. He claimed that state psychiatric hospitals "were, in large part,
warehouses for the idiosyncratic, the aged, the senile, the odd, and the
different." He had been strongly influenced by Thomas Szasz, who
denied that mental illness existed, and Petris approvingly quoted the
antipsychiatry thesis "that either we are all mad or none of us is mad."
In describing his role in passing the LPS legislation, Petris later wrote,
"We remembered that throughout history some of today's madmen can
become tomorrow's heroes."[10]

Nicholas Petris had also been influenced by theorists who claimed
that most psychiatric problems are caused by problems within the family. He noted that "the 'patient' is only one part of a family problem . . .
his bizarre behavior may be a very appropriate response to other family members."[11] Thus, Petris represented the many Californians, especially those in the Bay Area, who believed that most psychiatric

problems were caused by bad families. These were generally the same people who idealized the maltreated hero of Ken Kesey's *One Flew Over the Cuckoo's Nest* and who opposed all involuntary hospitalizations in the name of civil liberty. For such people, the LPS bill was a godsend to protect people's civil rights.

With the marriage of Southern California conservative John Birchers to northern California's liberal civil libertarians, passage of the Lanterman-Petris-Short Act grew more likely. State Senator Alan Short's name was added to ensure final passage, but he was not a major player. Public support for it was widespread, especially in the most conservative and liberal communities. In one public hearing on the proposed legislation, an elderly man from Santa Cruz recounted his seven months of involuntary psychiatric hospitalization, then "raised over his head a paperback copy of Ken Kesey's *One Flew Over the Cuckoo's Nest* and commended it to the subcommittee as 'the truth about the mental hospital.' The audience erupted in applause." Civil libertarians praised LPS, calling it "the Magna Carta of the mentally ill."[12] Groups that should have recognized the potentially disastrous consequences of the legislation were inexplicably silent. The 1,600-member California Psychiatric Association concerned itself primarily with the private practice of psychiatry and had little interest in the state hospitals. The 28,000-member California Association of Mental Health, always reluctant to criticize state politicians, timidly endorsed the legislation. In the absence of any effective opposition, LPS passed the state legislature in 1967 without a single dissenting vote and took effect on July 1, 1969.

It should be noted that the architects of LPS believed that virtually all individuals with psychiatric disorders were competent to make informed decisions regarding their need for treatment. Frank Lanterman labeled as "indefensible" the idea "that a mentally disturbed individual will not admit to being 'sick' and will not accept recommended treatment." Under LPS, all "will be free to decide whether they wish to enter or leave the hospitals." There would be no involuntary hospitalization, and this, said Lanterman, would free "thousands of persons from the 'tyranny of help' which has camouflaged for so many years the denial of liberty and basic human dignity."[13]

The Jonah Philosophy

It is apparent that Frank Lanterman and the other architects of LPS did not have individuals like Herb Mullin in mind when they crafted their legislation, nor did the public when supporting it. Although clearly psychotic, Mullin did not meet the "imminent dangerousness" criteria required for prolonged hospitalization and was thus released in November 1969. According to the new rules, it would be Mullin's choice, and his choice alone, whether to seek psychiatric help. He had been freed from the "tyranny of help."

Encouraged by his family, Mullin initially sought treatment at the Santa Cruz Mental Health Center. He took medication intermittently and attended group therapy sporadically. Like most community mental health centers of that era, the Santa Cruz Mental Health Center focused on helping people who had less severe psychiatric problems, often using Freudian principles and psychotherapy techniques to do so. Individuals with schizophrenia, like Herb Mullin, were of little interest to the mental health center staff, and conversely, the mental health center was of little interest to Mullin. Eventually he just stopped going, and the staff closed his case.

Without treatment, Mullin's life began a course that assumed an aura of inevitability. As he himself later remarked in response to why he had killed, "A rock doesn't make a decision while it's falling. It just falls."[14] Over the next several months, his behavior and lifestyle were erratic. He qualified for welfare payments because of his diagnosis of schizophrenia, but the payments carried no requirement that he seek treatment. He lived in a cheap Santa Cruz hotel and attempted to join a commune but was rejected because of his weird behavior. On one occasion, he propositioned a woman in the commune, and when she rejected him, "he picked up a hatchet and smashed it against the fireplace."[15] He spent a lot of his time studying astrology and numerology.

In June 1970, Mullin flew to Hawaii with a woman who had also been a patient at the mental health center. After spending two weeks at a Krishna Temple on Maui, the woman abandoned him. With no resources at hand, Mullin applied for voluntary admission to Maui Memorial Hospital, where he remained for a week. Diagnosed with schizophrenia, he professed nonviolence and behaved bizarrely, including walking out of the hospital to look for work while dressed in a hospital gown. He was again treated with Thorazine and Stelazine, improving enough that he could travel again. Hospitals in Hawaii regularly admitted psychiatrically ill individuals from the continental United States, and their primary goal was to get them back to the mainland. Mullin was thus escorted to the airport by police and put on a plane to San Francisco.

Mullin's parents met him at the airport and found him to be so disturbed that his father stopped at a telephone booth and called the police, asking them how he could have his son hospitalized. The police "told him they were powerless to force Herb to do anything if he had not committed a crime."[16] A week later, Mullin was arrested for strange behavior and involuntarily hospitalized at Santa Cruz County General Hospital for five days. He was suspected of being under the influence of drugs, which were found in his pocket. In court, Mullin shouted at the judge and demanded the legalization of marijuana and LSD. The drug charges were dropped when it was discovered that the drugs in his pocket were antipsychotic medications he had been given upon discharge from the hospital in Hawaii. He was released from jail and referred once again to the Santa Cruz Mental Health Center but could not be compelled to accept treatment.

During the next nine months, Mullin continued to lead a chaotic existence in Santa Cruz. He lived in a series of rented rooms, proselytized passersby on Pacific Avenue, changed the beneficiary of his life insurance policy to UNICEF, and spent ten days in jail for being drunk in public and resisting arrest. Like those of many individuals with schizophrenia, his symptoms fluctuated over time. During his better periods, he held a series of brief entry-level jobs and at one point applied for readmission to Cabrillo College but failed to follow through. His parents despaired; they explored every possible means to get treatment for their son but were consistently told that it was not possible under California's new law unless he voluntarily sought treatment himself.

* * *

In May 1971, Herb Mullin moved to San Francisco. He took up residence in a cheap hotel in the Tenderloin district, an area that was rapidly becoming overrun with overtly mentally ill persons in addition to its longstanding assortment of alcoholics and drug addicts. In the two years since the LPS Act had become law, the Bay Area had started to witness its effects. The Tenderloin district, like areas in other California cities, was gradually taking on the appearance of an open-air psychiatric ward.

San Francisco had a reputation for being remarkably tolerant of bizarre behavior, and Herb Mullin fit easily into the odd ambiance. He applied at a San Francisco gymnasium for boxing lessons, "speaking with a Spanish accent." A picture shows him "wearing a sombrero and reading a Bible as he sat watching professional boxers train." His sister also noted that, during a visit to her house, "he had a very heavy Spanish accent and wore a large, black hat." One acquaintance recalled Mullin standing in the kitchen one night for three or four hours, talking to God. Another said, "Sometimes it was impossible to understand what he was talking about. He'd jump from one subject to another with every sentence." Still another remembered Mullin as "very coherent" at some times but "obviously nuts" at others.[17]

Mullin had little contact with his family during these sixteen months, but what contact he had caused great distress. One day, in front of his elderly grandparents, he began taking off his clothes until he was escorted out of the house by his uncle. On another occasion, he walked into his uncle's home and said, "Uncle, I want to know if your balls are bigger than mine."[18] Mullin's parents continued to assess options for obtaining involuntary treatment for their son but were repeatedly told that it was not possible unless he could be proven to be imminently dangerous.

While living in San Francisco, still untreated, Herb Mullin became convinced that he was a prophet. He obsessed over the story of Jonah, cast overboard by his shipmates to appease God and thus calm the angry seas and save the others on board. Like many people, Mullin was convinced that a major earthquake in northern California was imminent. God had anointed him to prevent the earthquake by making human sacrifices. As he later explained at his trial, "We human beings, through the history of the world, have protected our continents from cataclysmic earthquakes by murder. In other words, a minor natural disaster avoids a major natural disaster." This, according to Mullin, was "the Jonah philosophy": people were assigned to die as sacrifices for others by singing "the die song." When asked to explain "the die song," he replied, "Just that. I'm telling you to die. I'm telling you to kill yourself, or be killed so that my continent will not fall off into the ocean . . . see, it's all based on reincarnation, this dies to protect my strata."[19]

Mullin was convinced of the reality of his belief system. When the death rate in the world goes up, he said, the number of natural disasters, such as earthquakes, goes down. He wrote to the United Nations and consulted public library reference books to prove his theory. How else could he explain the fact that his birthday and Albert Einstein's both fell on April 18, the same day on which the great San Francisco earthquake of 1906 had occurred? How else could he explain the many "cosmic emanations" he continued to receive?

By mid-September 1972, Mullin knew what he had to do. He accepted his mission reluctantly but gracefully. He referred to himself as a "scapegoat" and was convinced that in his reincarnation he would be properly rewarded, as Jonah had been returned to dry land from the whale's stomach. Murder was legally wrong but sometimes necessary for the greater good. He briefly contemplated suicide but decided that one death was not enough to avert the earthquake. More people would have to die, but how many? He returned to Santa Cruz to await instructions.

By the time Herb Mullin began murdering people, in October 1972, some Californians had started to wonder whether the LPS Act was producing an increase in violent acts. Among state officials, this was a sensitive issue. The question had been raised repeatedly in public hearings while the act was under consideration: Would the proposed legislation lead the state to release mentally ill individuals who might become violent? State officials had offered reassurance, citing studies showing that individuals with histories of mental illness had *lower* rates of violent behavior than the general population. This was true at the time, since most individuals with severe psychiatric disorders had been kept in hospitals until they were better. If the entire truth had been told, however, no data were available on what would happen if thousands of severely mentally ill persons were placed in community settings, many without their needed medications. California was to be the site of a grand experiment to find the answer.

Less than a month after returning to Santa Cruz, Herb Mullin began his slaughter. His first victim was Lawrence White, whom he spotted walking on an isolated road outside of town. As Mullin later described it, "He was like Jonah in the Bible, he was telling me, you know, telepathically, 'Hey, man, pick me up and throw me over the boat. Kill me so that others will be saved.'"[20] Mullin pulled his car to the side of the road, pretending to have car trouble. When White offered to help him, Mullin beat him to death with a baseball bat.

A week later, Mullin, driving past a Cabrillo College teacher he had known, heard the man say, "I want you to kill me somebody."[21] The next day, he picked up a hitchhiking Mary Guilfoyle and stabbed her to death with a hunting knife, then drove to a remote spot where he partially dissected her body and discarded it in the woods.

Nine days later, Mullin stopped at Saint Mary's Catholic Church in Los Gatos. It was All Souls Day, and he thought he should pray for the dead. When he entered the church, a voice told him to kill someone. Father Tomei was alone in the confessional; Mullin stabbed him to death, but only after the priest fought back fiercely.

Herb Mullin had murdered three people in less than three weeks. In retrospect, he expressed reservations about his actions, saying he knew it was wrong and didn't really want to kill people. During this period, he also applied to join the Coast Guard but failed the psychological examination. He then began discussions with a Marine Corps recruiter and, remarkably, in early January passed the requisite psychological exam. This was a testament both to the ability of some indi-

viduals with schizophrenia to look normal for brief periods and, presumably, to the desperation of recruiters in the late stages of the Vietnam War. Herb Mullin would have become a Marine in January 1973
had he not then refused to sign a copy of his criminal record, contend-
ing that it was inaccurate. The Marines thus withdrew their offer.

The rejections by the Coast Guard and the Marines greatly angered
Mullin. He became argumentative at home, and on January 19 his
father asked him to move elsewhere. He took an apartment in downtown Santa Cruz and plotted revenge against those he believed had
wronged him.

One such person was Jim Gianera, a friend from high school from
whom Mullin had bought some drugs during the early stages of his illness. He became convinced that Gianera was part of a conspiracy; as he
later explained, "Gianera spearheaded a movement to befuddle and
confuse me." On January 25, Mullin went to Gianera's former home,
where Kathy Francis and her two sons now lived. Kathy gave Mullin
the Gianeras' new address, and he went directly there and shot and
stabbed to death Gianera and his wife, Joan. Aware that Kathy Francis
could identify him, he returned to her home and shot and stabbed her
to death along with nine-year-old David and four-year-old Daemon.
These murders were made easier, he later said, by the fact that Kathy
had telepathically told him, "We are prepared to die. My children and
I don't mind being killed to prevent an earthquake."[22]

Two weeks later, Mullin was hiking in nearby Cowell State Park
when he came across four young men who were camping illegally.
He told them they were breaking the law and ordered them to leave.
They argued with him, and, as his later testimony would reveal, "he
received a telepathic message from the young men [that] it was all right
to kill them."[23] Mullin took out a revolver and shot them to death. The
boys had a rifle with them, and since they had no more use for it, he
took it.

Four days later, on February 13, 1973, Herb cut a load of firewood
to deliver to his mother, as she had requested. He then received a telepathic message to kill someone before delivering the wood. The stolen
rifle lay in the back seat. The first person Mullin saw was Fred Perez,

working in his yard. Mullin stopped his station wagon, rolled down the window, and killed him with a single shot. A woman across the street heard the gun's report and saw the station wagon driving away. She called the police, who spotted the vehicle ten minutes later and arrested Mullin. Perez was his thirteenth and last victim.

Herb Mullin's trial began in July 1973. From the outset, there was something disquieting about it. Day after day, descriptions of telepathic messages and human sacrifices stood in stark contrast to the descriptions of innocent people being murdered—bullet holes through the heads of two small boys playing with marbles, the dissected remains of a young woman. The randomness and senselessness of it hung in the courtroom air; by the end of the day, many viewers were left with a sense of emptiness.

The question in everyone's mind—why wasn't Mullin being treated?—was finally answered by Donald T. Lunde, an experienced forensic psychiatrist who testified for the defense. He explained that the problem was the Lanterman-Petris-Short Act:

> *Yes, the LPS. It was in effect certainly at this time. It is now impossible to commit somebody for a prolonged period in the state of California, even though you know, as was mentioned repeatedly here, that the patient is dangerous to himself or to others.*
>
> *The law provides very limited, very specific numbers of days that you can keep somebody. Beyond that, even though a person may continue to be obviously dangerous, he must be released.*[24]

The judge gently chided Lunde for oversimplifying the problem but then added, "I'm not going to quarrel with you because the Lanterman-Petris-Short Act is something I've quarreled with for a long time myself." Lunde then went on to describe the closing of state psychiatric hospitals, including "Mendocino, where Mullin was a patient," and added, "In other words, we have a situation where all the state hospitals are simply being closed down. So, as a practical matter, whether somebody is dangerous or not, there is no place to put him."[25]

There was never any doubt what the jury would decide, and when the verdict was announced on August 19, 1973, nobody appeared surprised. If Mullin was found not guilty by reason of insanity, he would have to be turned over to the California mental health authorities and hospitalized until he was well enough to be released. These were the same authorities who had discharged Mullin in the first place and who were discharging other patients as fast as they could, regardless of whether they were well enough to be released. The jury found Herbert Mullin guilty of ten counts of murder, the total number he was being tried for and for which the authorities had the strongest evidence, and the judge sentenced him to life in the California state prison system. Mullin's defense attorney correctly noted that "the jury did not want to find his client insane because the defendant could some day be released."[26] The jury chose its only logical option—put Mullin safely away for life in a place where the mental health authorities could not again release him.

The final commentary on the murders was provided by Kenneth Springer, the foreman of the Mullin jury. In a letter to Governor Ronald Reagan published on page one of the *Santa Cruz Sentinel* two days after the verdict, Springer wrote,

> *I hold the state executive and state legislative offices as responsible for these ten lives as I do the defendant himself—none of this need ever have happened.*
>
> *We had the awesome task of convicting one of our young valley residents of a crime that only an individual with a mental discrepancy could have committed. Five times prior to Mr. Mullin's arrest he was entered into mental facilities. At least twice it was determined that his illness could cause danger to lives of human beings. Yet in February and January of this year he was free to take the lives of Santa Cruz County residents.*
>
> *According to testimony at his trial, Herb Mullin could and did respond favorably to treatment of his mental illness. Yet, the laws of this state certainly*

prohibit officials from forcing continued treatment of his illness, and I have the impression that they, as a matter of fact, discourage continued treatment by state and county institutions.

In recent years, mental hospitals all over this state have been closed down in an economy move by the Reagan administration. Where do you think these mental institution patients who were in these hospitals went after their release? Do you suppose they went to private, costly mental hospitals? Or do you suppose they went to the ghettos of our large cities and to the remote hills of Santa Cruz County? . . .

I freely admit that I write this at a time when my emotions are not as clearly controlled as perhaps I would like them to be, but I cannot wait longer to impart to anyone who may read this my convictions that the laws surrounding mental illness in the State of California are wrong, wrong, wrong.[27]

4 | "The Odds Are Still in Society's Favor"

It would indeed be ironic if the Magna Carta of the mentally ill in California led to their criminal stigmatization and incarceration in jails and prisons, where little or no mental health treatment is provided.

MARC ABRAMSON, 1972

In 1973, at the time of Herb Mullin's trial, California was considered the standard-bearer for American psychiatry. In the 1950s, it had been one of the first states to make Thorazine, the new antipsychotic medication, available to all state psychiatric hospitals. During the 1960s, it had been the pacesetter in discharging patients from those hospitals. It had passed the Lanterman-Petris-Short Act (LPS) in 1967; a decade later, it would be said that "most state commitment statutes today are modeled after California's Lanterman-Petris-Short Act."[1] And then, most dramatically, Governor Ronald Reagan had announced in January 1973 that California would become the first state to close all its state psychiatric hospitals except for two used for the criminally insane. California was truly the leader in the deinstitutionalization movement. It would also be the leader in the disaster that followed.

Governor Reagan's proposal to shut down the state psychiatric hospitals was a proposal born of conviction. Like Frank Lanterman and Richard Nixon, Reagan was a product of Southern California's conservative anti–mental health culture. As an astute politician, Reagan was also aware that 71 percent of America's psychiatrists had voted Democratic in the 1964 presidential election and that almost two thousand of them had responded to a poll questioning the sanity of the Republican candidate, Barry Goldwater.[2] Reagan, understandably, was pleased to shut down anything associated with the psychiatric profession.

There is no indication that Reagan ever understood the need for psychiatric treatment. After he became president, tragedy struck the family of Reagan's friend and personal tax adviser, Roy Miller. The Millers went to church regularly, did not smoke or drink, and were described by the media as "the perfect American family." In 1981, the Millers' older son committed suicide after a "nervous breakdown" in college. Two years later, their younger son, diagnosed with schizophrenia, raped his mother and bludgeoned her to death.[3] Yet during those same years, the Reagan presidency undertook an unprecedented effort to reduce the number of psychiatrically disabled patients receiving federal support under the Supplemental Security Income (SSI) program, an effort that was subsequently reversed by a combination of public outrage and court action.[4] Even after being shot by John Hinckley, a delusional young man with untreated schizophrenia, Reagan publicly displayed no understanding of the underlying problem.

Ronald Reagan has frequently been called the father of deinstitutionalization in California, but technically this is not correct. The state hospitals had held over 37,000 patients in the mid-1950s; deinstitutionalization had begun under the Republican governor Goodwin Knight (1953–59) and continued under the Democratic governor Edmund "Pat" Brown (1959–67) before Reagan took office. The Lanterman-Petris-Short Act accelerated this process; within two years of its 1969 implementation, the number of state hospital patients had decreased from 18,831 to 12,671, and by 1973 the count had fallen to 7,000. Some 63 percent of the state's remaining psychiatric inpatients had been discharged within four years of passage of the new law, a result exactly in line with what the sponsors of LPS had intended.

In addition to promoting the discharge of patients, the implementation of LPS made it virtually impossible to get relapsed or newly ill psychiatric patients into hospitals, because of the need to demonstrate "imminent dangerousness." Between 1969 and 1978, there occurred a 99 percent decrease in the number of petitions for involuntary commitment filed with the courts. For the few patients who were involuntarily admitted, the average hospital stay decreased from 180 days to just 15.[5] When Herb Mullin was voluntarily admitted to Mendocino State Hospital in early 1969, the hospital was already being downsized and would subsequently be closed altogether. From 1970 to 1972, when Mullin was receiving occasional outpatient treatment in Santa Cruz, Agnews State Hospital, to which patients from Santa Cruz had previously been admitted, was also being shut down, as were hospitals in Stockton, Modesto, and DeWitt.

Governor Reagan's 1973 proposal to close California's state hospitals sparked an immediate controversy. As a result of LPS, communities throughout the state were already experiencing the effects of emptying the hospitals, and a vociferous public debate was underway. In San Jose in late 1971, the local newspaper decried the "mass invasion of mental patients," many of them homeless, discharged to downtown boarding-houses from nearby Agnews State Hospital as it was being closed.[6] The following year, the psychiatrist Marc Abramson published data showing that the number of mentally ill persons jailed in San Mateo County had doubled since the implementation of LPS.[7] In October 1970, John Frazier committed a highly publicized mass murder that some attributed to LPS and the closing of the hospitals. Frazier brutally murdered a prominent Santa Cruz eye surgeon, along with his wife, secretary, and two young sons, then threw their bodies into the swimming pool and set fire to the house. Frazier would later tell police that voices from God had told him "to seek vengeance on those who rape the environment." According to one account, "Frazier's wife and mother [had] tried desperately to obtain psychiatric treatment for him" but could not do so, because he had not yet demonstrated dangerousness.[8] The publicity surrounding such tragedies spurred members of the California legislature to decide it would be politically prudent to hold public hearings on Governor Reagan's proposal to close the remaining state psychiatric hospitals.

"The Slippage Factor"

The Senate Select Committee on Proposed Phaseout of State Hospital Services held eleven public hearings between May 18 and October 10, 1973, overlapping the period when Herbert Mullin was standing trial. The committee chairman was Alfred Alquist, a state senator from Santa Clara County. Other noteworthy members included George Deukmejian, who would be governor from 1983 to 1991; Alan Short, who was one of the authors of LPS; and Robert Lagomarsino, who would become a U.S. congressman and whose son was diagnosed with schizophrenia. The hearings repeatedly exposed problems with the mentally ill homeless, the mentally ill in jails, and homicides committed by mentally ill persons who were not receiving treatment.

Early in the hearings, Alquist highlighted the problem of "discharged patients . . . living in skid row, observed wandering aimlessly in the streets."[9] The vice mayor of San Jose described the "ghetto for the mentally ill and mentally retarded" composed of 1,800 patients from Agnews State Hospital who had been discharged to board and care homes clustered near the San Jose State University campus. "Ghettos of state hospital patients are forming in urban communities across the state," it was said. Asked to respond to these concerns, representatives of the State Department of Mental Health told the select committee that "under the Lanterman-Petris-Short Act . . . [the discharged patients] have the civil right to determine their actions for themselves. . . . [The] patients have elected to take up residence in some of these facilities." Department spokespersons referred to the large number of homeless mentally ill individuals who were receiving no psychiatric treatment as "the slippage factor."

For anyone in 1973 who truly wished to understand the origins of the increasing numbers of mentally ill homeless persons, studies were already available showing that these individuals were products of LPS, human hallmarks of its failure. Foremost among the researchers analyzing this problem was Richard Lamb, a forty-three-year-old Yale-trained psychiatrist then working for the San Mateo County Department of

Mental Health. Lamb was the first, and subsequently the foremost, critic of LPS, as he documented its failures for almost four decades. He also became a national leader decrying the consequences of inadequate commitment laws, including serving as chairman of the American Psychiatric Association's Task Force on the Homeless Mentally Ill.

As early as September 1969, Lamb publicly observed that most patients who were discharged from California's state hospitals were being inappropriately placed in rundown boarding homes that were no better, and in many cases worse, than the hospitals. The boarding homes, Lamb noted, "are in most respects like small, long-term state hospital wards isolated from the community." Patients in these facilities were frequently unsupervised, often unmedicated, and free to wander the streets. By 1973, the hospital discharge process had been publicly labeled as having changed the patients' venue "from back wards to back alleys." The following year, two more studies documented the reality that discharged patients "tend to be clustered into low-income areas in poor housing, suggesting a 'ghettoization' of ex-patients."[10]

The second major problem discussed during the 1973 senate hearings was the number of mentally ill persons in jail. A representative of the Santa Clara County Sheriff's Department testified at the hearings that the problem of mentally ill inmates had become "probably ten times larger" during the preceding decade: "We have created a special ward in our County Jail to house just the individuals that presently have such a mental condition." The Los Angeles County sheriff estimated that "between 40 and 50 percent of the 8,500 Los Angeles County inmates are in need of urgent psychiatric care." He further predicted that if the state hospitals continued to be closed, "the effect of such phaseout on law enforcement would be manifested in an apparent higher crime rate." The sheriff of San Joaquin County testified about the situation since LPS had gone into effect: "The courts and a number of other agencies in the community, including us I'm sad to tell you, are interpreting bizarre or incoherent or unusual behavior as criminality. . . . A good deal of mental illness is now being interpreted as criminality."

Dr. James Stubblebine, the director of the California Department of

Mental Health, was the principal spokesperson for the state during the hearings. He was a psychiatrist and devout believer that CMHCs should replace the state hospital system, which he described as "an unnecessary relic of the past and, like many antiquities, it is extremely expensive." Stubblebine played to the fiscal conservatives by focusing especially on the potential cost savings that the government would realize if state hospitals were closed:

> *We believe that a comprehensive local mental health program that functions effectively is, in fact, an inexpensive health delivery system when compared to the traditional method of using distant state hospitals for acute psychiatric care. . . . The states and taxpayers are probably saving money by using the community mental health system.*

Stubblebine enthusiastically supported LPS, which, he said, would result in "the virtual disappearance of [psychiatric] commitment except for a handful of patients, mostly the elderly with severe chronic brain syndromes."[11]

When asked to respond to allegations that the implementation of LPS was increasing the number of mentally ill persons in California's jails, Stubblebine responded that "specific information is not available which would indicate that more discharged patients are going into the jails." This statement was untrue. At the time Dr. Stubblebine testified, three studies published in 1971 and 1972 were already available with this "specific information," and during 1973 an additional study came out.[12]

Foremost among these studies was one by Marc Abramson, in San Mateo County, who in 1972 had reported that, in the year following implementation of LPS, criminal complaints had increased 36 percent and mentally ill individuals judged incompetent to stand trial had increased 100 percent. Abramson contended that "as a result of LPS, mentally disordered persons are being increasingly subjected to arrest and criminal prosecution." Because it was so difficult to commit persons to psychiatric hospitals under LPS, he added, police "regard arrest and booking into jail as a more reliable way of securing involuntary detention of mentally disordered persons." Abramson also quoted the published view of a prison psychiatrist who said, "We are literally drowning in patients. . . . The crisis stems from recent changes in the mental health laws. . . . Many more men are being sent to prison who have serious mental problems."[13]

The third, and by far most controversial, problem discussed during the 1973 hearings was the possible increase in homicides committed by mentally ill individuals. The potential for this increase had been raised in public hearings prior to the passage of LPS, and it was a politically sensitive issue both for state legislators and for officials in the State Department of Mental Health. Nobody wanted to be associated with legislation that led to more homicides. Chairman Alquist, in the opening session, asked Dr. Stubblebine about reports of "violent crimes committed by people who have been committed [to hospitals] for previous violent crimes because of insanity, and yet after a period of a year or two were released as sane and able to return to society, and immediately go out and commit another violent crime." Senator Deukmejian similarly alluded to "a number of very serious kinds of events including multiple murders and the like."

At the time of the hearings, several cases of psychiatrically related multiple homicides in California were in the headlines. In the months leading up to the hearings, Mary Maloney had decapitated her infant daughter and year-old son. Her husband had tried to have her psychiatrically hospitalized prior to the crime, but she had not met the LPS criteria for dangerousness. Charles Soper had killed his wife, three children, and himself two weeks after being discharged from Camarillo State Hospital because he failed to qualify as "imminently dangerous." In April 1973, one month before the start of the hearings, Edmund Kemper had been arrested after he bludgeoned his mother to death, then strangled her friend who came to visit. Kemper was also charged with the murders of six female hitchhikers. His case was widely publicized throughout California when it was disclosed that eight years earlier, at age fifteen, Kemper had shot his grandmother and grandfather to death because "he tired of their company." He was subsequently hospitalized until he turned twenty-one, in 1969, the same year LPS took effect. Kemper had then been released without any follow-up psychiatric treatment.[14]

The case of Hebert Mullin, whose trial was taking place at the same time as the hearings, loomed largest over the proceedings. When Chairman Alquist asked witnesses, as he did on several occasions, "Have we gone too far in protecting individuals' civil liberties?," it was Mullin who initially came to mind for most observers.

On October 9, 1973, Kenneth Springer, the foreman of the Mullin jury, testified before the California Senate Select Committee. Two months before, he had published his criticism of Governor Reagan and other state officials after Mullin's trial. At the October hearings, he took up where he had left off. "The reason why Mr. Mullin couldn't receive continued hospitalization and treatment," Springer testified, was that LPS "makes it impossible to commit a person, even though one knows he is dangerous, for a prolonged period of time." Springer ridiculed the assumption that severely mentally ill persons would volunteer to be treated, arguing that only "sane persons volunteer for medical treatment." Springer likened the effects of LPS to "releasing known killers from our prisons, arming them, and then turning them loose on society." "The closing of our mental hospitals," he added, "is, in my opinion, insanity itself." Finally, Springer asked, "Was Herb Mullin any more responsible for those 13 lives than those public officials who perpetuate this insane law that allowed him to be free to kill 13 people?"

The task of rebutting allegations that LPS was increasing the number of homicides in California fell to Dr. Stubblebine and his deputy, Dr. Andrew Robertson, from the Department of Mental Health.

Stubblebine stated on May 18, early in the hearings, "I know that there are a lot of people who are concerned about this issue and I have staff working on the question . . . [of] how many people who were formerly diagnosed as mentally ill do indeed commit violent crimes." By the time Stubblebine returned to testify again, on October 9, he had received the report of his department's study, but he did not mention it to the committee. The study found that, among 6,623 individuals who had been convicted of murder, manslaughter, or felony assault in California in 1971, 12 percent had been previously treated in state psychiatric hospitals or community mental health programs. The rate of such crimes committed by individuals discharged from the hospitals, according to the state data, was seven times higher than the rate for the general population. The results of this study were never published; a copy, however, was obtained by Larry Sosowsky, a graduate student at the University of California at Berkeley, and some of the data were later included in Sosowsky's publication on this problem.[15]

It was left to Dr. Andrew Robertson, Stubblebine's deputy, to deliver a definitive, and most remarkable, rebuttal to allegations that LPS was increasing homicides in California. Testifying before the select committee, Robertson explained,

> It [LPS] has exposed us as a society to some dangerous people; no need to argue about that. People whom we have released have gone out and killed other people, maimed other people, destroyed property; they have done many things of an evil nature without their ability to stop and many of them have immediately thereafter killed themselves. That sounds bad, but let's qualify it . . . the odds are still in society's favor, even if it doesn't make patients innocent nor the guy who is hurt or killed feel any better.[16]

"America's Newest Mental Institution"

In 1972, as California was emptying its state psychiatric hospitals, a county mental health official presciently observed,

> The reorganization of the state hospitals can be seen as an experiment in the field of community psychiatry. . . . Certainly all the proposed changes will not pan out; certainly not all change is progress. However, the disappointments can be instructive and maturing if we make them so. At this point we cannot know what will happen. We can only work, observe and grow.[17]

It was a warning that those in government should have heeded. Instead, they had launched deinstitutionalization in California like a large ship, with bands playing and much public fanfare. Once it was in the water, its designers were determined to see it sail. Beneath its waterline, however, were three large holes in the shape of the letters L, P, and S; the outcome of the voyage was foreordained.

For the homeless, the situation described during the 1973 select committee hearings became progressively worse. Many discharged patients were placed in rundown boardinghouses with little or no psychiatric supervision. As these individuals stopped taking their medication and wandered away from their shabby accommodations, observers noted an increase in the numbers of mentally ill homeless persons on the streets. By the mid-1980s, California State Assemblyman Bruce Bronzan estimated that there were "between 20,000 and 50,000 adults who are chronically mentally ill and may be homeless," a situation Bronzan labeled "morally unacceptable and just unbelievable." Richard Lamb added, "Probably nothing more graphically illustrates the problems of deinstitutionalization than the shameful and incredible phenomenon of the homeless mentally ill."[18]

The problem was most visible in the cities. In Los Angeles, a 1985 study reported, 30 to 50 percent of all homeless persons were seriously mentally ill, and they were being seen in "ever increasing numbers." The study noted, "They are defenseless and frequently victimized . . . beaten, robbed and raped daily . . . [and] often eat garbage and sleep in alley ways." The study concluded that homeless mentally ill persons "are in part the product of the deinstitutionalization movement" and that the "new liberalized Mental Health laws [making] involuntary psychiatric treatment almost impossible . . . the 'Streets' have become 'The Asylums' of the 80s."[19]

Other studies confirmed these findings. A 1988 study of 529 Los Angeles street persons, for example, reported that 44 percent had had a previous psychiatric hospitalization; among that group, 28 percent obtained "some food" from garbage cans and 8 percent utilized garbage cans as their "primary food source." Another study of mentally ill street persons found that 79 percent of them had been previously psychiatrically hospitalized, 74 percent had been arrested at least once, 38 percent "had a history of serious violence against persons," and 30 percent "were not only disorganized but too paranoid to accept help." For such individuals, the authors concluded, "homelessness was not primarily a housing problem."[20]

For families that helplessly watched their ill family member live on the streets, deinstitutionalization had brought about a special kind of hell. One father, writing in the *Los Angeles Times*, noted,

> *I am financially able and willing to pay for psychiatric care and hospitalization for my daughter; she does not have to be the Skid Row inhabitant that she is. . . . She denies any illness and prefers to live on the streets. . . . The mental health law . . . makes impossible the provision of mental health therapy or even control if the sick person rejects such and asserts his or her civil rights.*[21]

In San Francisco, an estimated 40 percent of the homeless population was severely mentally ill. Among their ranks were well-educated individuals, such as a man with schizophrenia who was a graduate of Stanford University and Stanford Law School and who, according to his father, "lives in the streets and we believe he has been sleeping in the bushes several blocks from our home. . . . He needs hospitalization and custodial care, but we can't seem to get any help for him without violating his 'civil rights.' It is very painful for all of us." When a San Francisco television station ran a series on the homeless problem in 1989, it put up posters throughout the city saying, "You are now walking through America's newest mental institution." By 1990, a newspaper poll in San Francisco reported homelessness to be the city's number one problem for "the overwhelming majority of San Franciscans."[22]

A Bag Lady in San Francisco

In 1997, Shannon Morgan was a sixty-seven-year-old bag lady in San Francisco. She had previously graduated from college, obtained a medical degree from Cornell, and completed a residency in ophthalmology.

She had married and had two children. Then she became sick, like her sister who also had schizophrenia. For one year, she lived under a pine tree in northern California. As a homeless person in San Francisco, she wandered the streets "toting a 40-pound knapsack on her back, hauling her belongings in a luggage cart." The director of the Coalition for Homelessness in San Francisco was quoted as saying, "We are seeing more women in general, senior women in particular. It's inhumane."

J. H. Lee, "From the Ivy League to homelessness and mentally ill in San Francisco," Associated Press, October 12, 1997.

By the late 1990s, most Californians had concluded that something had indeed gone drastically wrong with the state mental health system. In 1998, San Francisco's homeless population had climbed to an estimated 16,000, of which more than 6,000 were mentally ill. Mayor Willie Brown called it "the most complex problem" he had faced as mayor. The *San Francisco Chronicle* described the issue as a "cancer on This City's soul." Across the Bay, the historically ultra-tolerant Berkeley was fed up also, and the city council passed ordinances restricting the rights of the homeless. A spokesperson said, "On any night, there are 1,000 to 1,200 people sleeping on the streets of Berkeley. Half of them are deinstitutionalized mentally ill people. It's like a mental ward on the streets."[23]

"Who's Going to Protect Paul from Paul?"

At the age of forty-four, Paul had lived for months in a waist-high space under a railroad bridge in Sacramento. He slept on the dirt amid rotting garbage and rats. He exhibited overtly psychotic behavior, such as walking through neighborhoods with his arms extended and "fecal matter in his hands." When he was seen in an emergency room, his feet were covered with mold. All attempts to persuade him to accept psychiatric treatment were to no avail. A Sacramento police officer, commenting on California's commitment laws, said, "It's gone too far one way. Who's going to protect Paul from Paul? We're going to go out one day and find him dead."

P. Hoge, "Bill aims to give aid even if it's spurned,"
Sacramento Bee, April 30, 2000.

"The Mad and the Bad"

The second indicator of California's failed deinstitutionalization program was the rising number of mentally ill individuals in the jails and prisons. Marc Abramson had predicted this in 1972, and over the next decade multiple studies confirmed LPS's contribution to the increase. In Los Angeles, Richard Lamb and his colleagues published four studies documenting in detail the continuing "criminalization of the mentally ill." In San Francisco, a study of five hundred mentally ill persons who had committed crimes, half misdemeanors and half felonies, reported that most of the crimes "derive from acute psychotic processes. . . . [A]t the time of arrest, 94 percent were not involved in any outpatient program. . . . The law is so strict and inflexible that it disallows the treatments that might be effective."[24]

During the 1980s and 1990s, the full effect of LPS on California's criminal justice system became manifest. Between 1980 and 1993 in San Francisco County, jail psychiatric services increased 99 percent. In Santa Clara County, the use of the jail psychiatric unit doubled between 1986 and 1991. By 1995, it was reported that 28 percent of the prisoners in the Sacramento County Jail were on psychiatric medications. And in Los Angeles, "15 to 17 percent of Los Angeles County Jail inmates—approximately 3,400 prisoners—were classified as mentally ill." By then, this jail had become, de facto, the largest mental institution in the United States. When Los Angeles County Corrections Chief Charles Jackson was asked in a television interview, "So what do you run here? Do you run a jail or do you run a mental institution?," he responded, "I run both."[25]

The flood of mentally ill individuals into California's jails and prisons in the closing decades of the twentieth century was a major factor in the overcrowding of these institutions. Exposés, investigations, and reports became as predictable as the seasons. As one investigation noted, "We observed cell after cell crowded with inmates who were psychotic or severely depressed and getting worse. . . . Overcrowding throughout the jail system has reached its worse level in years, with inmates sleeping on the floors, in the mess hall and in the chapels. . . ."[26]

Among corrections officials, it has been known for many years that "the mad and the bad don't mix," especially not in overcrowded conditions. Psychotic inmates often act bizarrely, such as those in the Alameda County Jail who tried "to escape by smearing themselves with their own feces and flushing themselves down the toilet." When similar behavior affects other inmates, the results can be tragic:

- In the Los Angeles County Jail two inmates . . . "beat to death Steven Pendergast, 33, who had recently been released from a mental hospital. Apparently Mr. Pendergast was mumbling to himself, which upset his bunkmates."

Psychotic inmates also find it difficult to understand or follow jail rules:

- In the Los Angeles County Jail a 27-year-old man with paranoid schizophrenia was severely beaten by guards, causing permanent brain damage. He had been "violating jail rules requiring inmates to remain silent, place their hands in their pockets, and keep their shirts tucked in" while waiting in the cafeteria line.[27]

Suicide is another consequence of putting mentally ill people in jail, both because many suffer from depression when they are admitted and because incarceration exacerbates depression. A study of inmates who attempted suicide in the Sacramento County Jail found that "more than half were experiencing hallucinations or delusions at the time of the attempt" and "more than 75% had histories of previous mental health treatment."[28]

For corrections officials, one of the most discouraging aspects of their work is seeing the same mentally ill individuals repeatedly cycling through the jail system. For the Los Angeles police unit that specializes in psychiatric evaluations, it was found that, in 1990, 65 percent of individuals evaluated "had been seen in the unit before, with 31 percent having been in police custody ten or more times." In Orange County during 1998 alone, 300 mentally ill offenders were rearrested three times, and 119 others were rearrested four times.[29] Such recurring penal pilgrimages have contributed to overcrowded jails and wasted police resources. From approximately the mid-1980s onward, most severely mentally ill individuals in California could count on spending more of their lives in jails than in psychiatric hospitals.

The LPS statute also profoundly affected police officers on the streets of California. Between 1987 and 1993, calls to the Los Angeles Police Mental Evaluation Unit more than quadrupled, from 12,613 to 54,737. Police were reported to spend more time on calls for "mental health crisis" than on calls for robberies. One officer described having picked up the same woman and taken her to the hospital sixteen times for lying down in the street: "Every time they just medicate her and send her home." LPS had permanently changed the nature of police work from primarily crime fighting to a mix of crime fighting and social work.[30]

The biggest psychiatric problem for law enforcement officers, however, was knowing how to handle psychotic individuals who were threatening violence. In some cases, officers were killed in such confrontations. More often, though, the confrontation ended with the mentally ill person dead. In Ventura County, with a population of 700,000, police killed 32 people in the ten-year period between 1992 and 2001; more than half of them (56 percent) were mentally ill.[31]

"We Do Grave Danger"

The third indicator that California's grand experiment had failed was the increase in episodes of violence, including homicides, committed by mentally ill individuals. In 1974, less than a year after state officials had assured the select committee that discharged patients would not be unduly violent, Larry Sosowsky released the preliminary results of his study. He had investigated 301 individuals from San Mateo County who had been discharged from Napa State Hospital after LPS had been implemented. Some 41 percent of them had been arrested following their release, and that could not be explained by their previous criminal behavior. As Sosowsky observed, "Patients who entered the hospital without a criminal record were subsequently arrested about three times as often as the average [San Mateo] citizen and five times as often for violent crimes."[32]

The *San Francisco Chronicle*, commenting on Sosowsky's findings, noted that 59 percent of the released patients had received no psychiatric care whatsoever after returning to San Mateo County. By way of explanation, the chief of the county's Mental Health Services said that "once released from state mental hospitals, former patients are under no compulsion to seek or accept psychiatric aid." State Senator H. L. Richardson, appearing with Sosowsky at a news conference, called for a "serious investigation of the current state's policy of turning most mentally ill Californians out of large state-run hospitals and back to communities, which seem apparently unable or unwilling to help them." Sosowsky concluded that "we may well be faced with the unpleasant fact that the emerging new legal relationship between the state and the mentally ill . . . may well incur a heretofore unassessed social cost—more crime and violence in the nation's communities."[33]

The issue had been clearly joined—how much additional violent crime were Californians willing to accept in order to protect the civil rights of patients with psychiatric illnesses? Stephen Morse, at the University of Southern California School of Law, argued in the *Wall Street Journal* that "our society ought to be willing to absorb a certain amount of violent behavior in order to preserve civil liberties for all of us." Sosowsky, by contrast, argued that it was possible to reconcile "the current concern for civil liberties and the expectation that public safety will be maintained," and he advocated the modification of LPS. "We do grave danger," he added," by averting our gaze from this persistent dilemma or taking comfort from the fact that the social cost is not greater."[34]

Over the next three decades, violent behavior, including homicides by individuals with severe psychiatric disorders, became more and more commonly reported in California. Some of the incidents were highly publicized.

- **1976:** Edward Allaway shot and killed seven people in the library at Cal State Fullerton. He had been diagnosed with paranoid schizophrenia and hospitalized five years earlier. He had delusions that people were trying to hurt him.
- **1988:** Dorothea Montalvo, who ran a Sacramento rooming house, was accused of murdering at least seven elderly boarders and burying their bodies in her yard. She had previously been diagnosed with schizophrenia and, at the time of the slaying, was on probation for drugging and robbing previous boarders.
- **1993:** Linda Scates drove her car into a pack of eight bicyclists, killing one and permanently injuring another. Voices had commanded her to "kill the demons." Six years earlier, she had been diagnosed with schizophrenia and involuntarily hospitalized for trying to run over a neighbor with her car.[35]

Although there is no federal or state central registry that keeps track of such episodes, the Treatment Advocacy Center, with which this author is associated, in Arlington, Virginia, does so by collecting media accounts. Hundreds of such records give a definite impression that violent episodes have become more common in California in recent years. That would not be surprising, for several reasons, one being the continuing increase in California's population. As was noted in chapter 1, the deinstitutionalization movement did not select random patients for discharge; the least sick went out first and the sickest last of all. Finally, there is a general impression in California that outpatient psychiatric services have substantially deteriorated in the past decade. Much of this decline can be attributed to the increased use of managed care and other for-profit companies to manage outpatient services.

For all of these reasons, one could expect that episodes of violent behavior in California by individuals with severe psychiatric disorders would have continued to increase—and they did. The following are a representative sample of cases from 1999 to 2001.

- **1999:** Steven Abrams, diagnosed with schizophrenia, intentionally drove his car onto a preschool playground, killing two young children in Costa Mesa. He believed that by doing so he would stop the government from beaming voices into his brain. He had been previously psychiatrically hospitalized and for five years had spoken of killing children.

- **1999:** Julie Rodriguez, diagnosed with schizophrenia, drove her car into the Sacramento River, killing herself and her two children. Her family had tried unsuccessfully to have her committed on numerous occasions, including evaluations by mental health professionals, police, and child protective services.

- **2000:** Marie West, diagnosed with bipolar disorder, intentionally ran over and killed an elderly man in Van Nuys. She had had nineteen previous psychiatric hospitalizations and had been released six days prior to the crime.

- **2000:** Gabriel Estrada, diagnosed with schizophrenia, stabbed to death his brother's neighbor in Santa Ana. Estrada had been hospitalized several times. Social workers and police had recently twice evaluated him at the request of his family but said they could do nothing because of the restrictive LPS laws.

- **2001:** David Attias, diagnosed with bipolar disorder, drove his car onto a Santa Barbara sidewalk, killing four people and injuring nine. He then got out of his car and announced that he was the "angel of death." Five years earlier, he had been hospitalized after trying to strangle his sister.

- **2001:** Scott Thorpe, diagnosed with paranoid schizophrenia, killed three people and attempted to kill three others at a restaurant and mental health clinic in Nevada City. Thorpe had previously threatened clinic staff and was known to be potentially dangerous but had not met the dangerousness requirements needed for involuntary commitment.

One of the people Scott Thorpe killed was Laura Wilcox, who was temporarily working at the mental health center as a receptionist. Shortly after the murders, Laura Wilcox's father said, "We strongly believe that the civil rights of mentally ill [persons] should be respected and protected, but civil rights are not absolute." His daughter, he added, had been permanently deprived "of her most fundamental civil right, the right to life."[36]

California Today

Governor Reagan's 1973 proposal to close all California state hospitals except two facilities for the criminally insane was ultimately rejected. Following the Senate Select Committee hearings, a bill was passed by the legislature prohibiting Reagan from closing additional hospitals without the consent of the legislature. Reagan vetoed the bill, but the legislature overrode his veto. It was the only veto override of Reagan's governorship and the first override of any California governor in twenty-seven years.

Despite this new legislation, the State Department of Mental Health continued to close state hospital beds without entirely closing the hospitals. In 1959, there had been 37,500 beds. When LPS was implemented in 1969, there were still almost 19,000. By 2003, the number had fallen to 4,275, three-quarters of which were meant for patients who had been judged to be criminally insane and thus mandated to involuntary hospitalization by the courts. It is important to note that the 37,500 state hospital beds available in 1955 were for a state population of 13.2 million—1 bed for every 352 people. In 2003, the 4,275 beds served a population of 35.5 million—1 bed for every 8,304 people. If the same number of state psychiatric beds available in 1955, proportional to population, had been available in 2003, they would have numbered 100,852. To be sure, many of the people who might have occupied one of those beds are better off than they would have been if they had still been in the hospital. They live with their families, in boarding homes run by caring operators, or on their own. Some are able to hold jobs, at least part-time, and most have a social life and the freedom to come and go as they please. Most of those who do well continue to take medication to control the symptoms of their illness and recognize the necessity for doing so. For these individuals, deinstitutionalization has indeed been a positive development. For the others, it has been, to varying degrees, a disaster.

The problem of mentally ill homeless persons in California is greater today than it has ever been and is apparently continuing to grow. In San Francisco, there are endless discussions about what to do; public programs such as Operation Scrub Down (removing from the streets the shopping carts used by homeless persons) and Care Not Cash (providing food and housing in place of welfare payments) have had little effect. The magnitude of the city's problem received national attention in 2003 when a prominent psychiatrist, attending the annual meeting of the American Psychiatric Association, was knocked unconscious by a mentally ill homeless man as she walked down the street; the irony of the attack was widely publicized.

A 2005 study reported that, in San Diego, among all patients receiving public psychiatric services, 20 percent of those with schizophrenia and 17 percent of those with bipolar disorder were homeless as their "modal living situation."[37] In Los Angeles in 2005, Mayor Antonio Villaraigosa visited skid row and commented, "I mean that almost looked like Bombay or something, except with more violence. There is no place [in the city] where the chaos and degradation are as pronounced. You see a complete breakdown of society." The *Los Angeles Times* called the skid row scene "a human catastrophe unfolding" and concluded that "laws intended to protect the rights of . . . mentally ill people are well-intended but inhumane." In 2007, Governor Arnold Schwarzenegger proposed abolishing a $55 million state program to help homeless persons with serious mental illnesses; it appeared that the state had given up efforts to solve the problem.[38]

"A Sadly Routine Occurrence"

In May 2005, Marina Brandt died of pneumonia an hour after arriving at the Union Rescue Mission on Los Angeles's skid row. Her only iden- tification was a plastic armband from the hospital from which she had just been discharged. The daughter of an engineer, Brandt had grown up with a swimming pool in her yard, been an A student in high school, and attended UCLA before developing schizophrenia.

Over the ensuing twenty-five years, Brandt suffered the conse- quences of California's chaotic treatment system, the product of dein- stitutionalization and LPS. She was frequently homeless and said to be "easy prey for sexual abuse." She abused drugs and attacked her sis- ter "with two kitchen knives." Despite multiple brief hospitalizations and large sums of money spent by her family trying to stabilize her, she resisted all treatment efforts. According to the newspaper, her death was said to be "a sadly routine occurrence on skid row."

C. M. DiMassa, "Falling through the cracks," Los Angeles Times, December 24, 2005.

The presence of mentally ill persons in California's jails and prisons has also grown progressively worse. A 1999 state report concluded that 11 percent of the county jail population and 20 percent of the state prison population were "severely mentally ill." In Los Angeles, a 2003 study "found that 28 percent of male and 31 percent of female arrestees had either a significant history of mental illness or were manifesting symptoms of mental illness at the time of arrest." For every county in California for which records are available, the county jail now holds more severely mentally ill people than any hospital in that county.[39]

The consequences of this state of affairs have been predictable. In 2002, California jail suicides reached a record level. Exposés of jail con- ditions for mentally ill inmates have been published so regularly that they are no longer news. A 2005 account of the San Mateo County Jail, for example, described nineteen inmates who had been waiting for beds at Napa State Hospital, some for as long as nine months. One "said he thinks that perhaps he is in Italy being held by the mob." Another "lies curled up naked in a pool of urine."[40]

Conditions in the state prisons, where 20 percent of the 172,000 inmates are mentally ill, are even worse. In 2005, a U.S. judge ordered a federal takeover of the prisons because of medical "incompetence and at times outright depravity." In 1993, California spent $21 million for psychiatric care in state prisons; by 2003, the figure had reached $245 million.[41] The Department of Corrections advertises itself as "one of the largest providers of mental health care in California." In fact, it probably *is* the largest.

Homicides and other violent acts committed by mentally ill individuals have also continued to plague California. In the thirty-five years following implementation of the LPS Act, a total of 94,382 homicides were reported in California. If severely mentally ill persons were responsible for only 5 percent of these, a conservative estimate based on studies reviewed in chapter 9, that would be 4,719 homicides. This number is for completed homicides only and not for other types of violence, including rapes, assaults, and attempted homicides. When calculating the true cost of failing to treat individuals with severe psychiatric disorders, one must include the effects of all violent crimes.

Most of these homicides and other acts of violence are never publicized. Periodically, however, high-profile cases become page one stories for a day or two, flashing like meteors across public consciousness before disappearing.

- **October 2005, San Francisco:** Lashuan Harris, diagnosed with schizophrenia, killed her three young sons by dropping them into San Francisco Bay in response to voices telling her to feed them to the sharks. Ms. Harris had not been taking her medication and had recently been turned down for admission to a psychiatric hospital.[42]
- **February 2006, Goleta:** Jennifer San Marco, who apparently had untreated paranoid schizophrenia, shot to death a former neighbor, six workers at a postal plant where she used to work, and herself.[43]
- **March 2006, Pismo Beach:** Lawrence Woods, suffering from paranoid schizophrenia, killed two people, injured two others, and

then killed himself in a Denny's restaurant. He was well known to be paranoid and "thought neighbors were ganging up on him." One neighbor had called county mental health workers to request help for him but was told "they couldn't help until Woods did something to warrant their help or asked for help himself."[44]

Such tragedies have become so common in California that the deputy district attorney in San Joaquin County publicly complained to a local newspaper that "he has prosecuted too many murderers with previously diagnosed mental health problems and is tired of it." In the preceding two years, he had personally prosecuted various severely mentally ill individuals who had bludgeoned to death two men, stabbed to death a nine-year-old, decapitated an eighteen-month-old, and set fire to a trailer, killing a man.[45] The number of homicides committed by mentally ill individuals does not, of course, include the number of mentally ill individuals who are themselves killed by law enforcement officials. As was noted previously, data available from Ventura County for 1992 to 2001 showed that eighteen mentally ill individuals were killed by police.[46]

California's Continuing Mistakes

The sad case of Kanuri Qawi suggests that California authorities have not learned from their mistakes. Previously known as Kenny Washington, Qawi was diagnosed with paranoid schizophrenia in 1990, when he severely assaulted a woman walking down an Oakland street, accusing her of having caused the war in Vietnam. For the next fourteen years, he was in and out of psychiatric hospitals and prisons, accumulating multiple additional charges, including the stalking of women. He consistently denied he was sick and refused medication. In 2000, he petitioned the court for the right to refuse medication; the case ultimately went to the California Supreme Court, which in 2004 upheld his request by a vote of 6 to 1. Under the ruling, individuals like Qawi can be involuntarily medicated only after a court hearing that establishes them to be dangerous or incompetent. In February 2005,

Qawi was released from the hospital and not required to take medication.

In the fall of 2006, in Alameda, Qawi was charged with the murder of John Milton, who shared his apartment. Milton had been stabbed seven times, then left for several days in the apartment until the smell of decaying flesh alerted authorities.

J. Richman, "Forcible medication of ex-cons limited,"
Alameda Times-Star, January 6, 2004; S. Gold and
L. Romney, "A profound but controversial effect,"
Los Angeles Times, March 16, 2007.

Many people in California have known that the state's mental health system, in general, and its commitment laws, in particular, have failed. Even Frank Lanterman, the L in LPS, eventually said, "I wanted the LPS act to help the mentally ill. I never meant for it to prevent those who need care from receiving it. The law has to be changed."[47] Such sentiment gave rise to periodic calls for revision of LPS and for reform of the treatment system. No serious attempt to do so, however, took place until Mike Bowers, a man with paranoid schizophrenia, issued a dramatic wake-up call to California legislators.

Bowers had a fifteen-year history of psychiatric hospitalizations and incarcerations, although he did well intermittently when he took his medication. When psychotic, he believed he was "King" of a "New World Order" and sought public recognition for his imagined accomplishments. In January 2001, he was employed as a truck driver but had stopped taking his medication. Driving an eighteen-wheel tractor-trailer, he picked up a full load of condensed milk in Modesto for delivery to South Dakota. Instead, he headed for downtown Sacramento, where, "blaring his horn and running at speeds of up to 70 mph," he drove his truck up some steps and into the side door of the capitol building. The truck knocked down the wall of a senate hearing room and exploded, killing Bowers instantly. The governor and state legislators, meeting elsewhere in the building at the time, hastily left. The next morning, in a room immediately above the burned-out truck, which still contained Bowers's body, a previously scheduled hearing was held on the inadequacy of medical and psychiatric care in the state's prisons.[48]

Mike Bowers's dramatic entry into the California capitol occurred just six days after Scott Thorpe, also diagnosed with schizophrenia, had killed Laura Wilcox and two others in nearby Nevada City. The killings attracted an unusual amount of media attention because Wilcox was an especially promising young woman, a candidate for student body president at Haverford College who had been home for the holidays and was merely filling in for a sick employee when she was killed. A bill to amend the state's commitment laws had been languishing in legislative committees for months. After Bowers's truck hit the capitol building, the bill suddenly became a priority, was christened "Laura's Law" in memory of the deceased young woman, and was signed into law by Governor Gray Davis. The new law allowed, for the first time, court-ordered outpatient treatment for people with serious psychiatric disorders who refuse to take medication and are potentially dangerous. The law was aimed directly at people like Mike Bowers and Scott Thorpe.

Passing legislation and implementing it, however, are two different things and sometimes only distantly related. Although Laura's Law was passed, opponents of the legislation added a provision stating that funds for existing psychiatric services could not be used to implement it. This essentially vitiated the legislation, and it consequently has been little used. Opposition to any kind of involuntary psychiatric treatment remains strong in California, led by the same unholy alliance that got LPS passed in 1967. On the one hand are fiscal conservatives who oppose most state expenditures, especially those concerning mental health matters. On the other hand are liberals and civil libertarians who view any involuntary treatment as illegitimate governmental intrusion. Today, as in 1967, this conservative-liberal coalition continues to control mental health policy in California.

Regarding costs, fiscal conservatives are correct that, on first glance, treating people with mental illnesses appears to be more expensive than not treating them. In Los Angeles in 2004, the cost per day for a person in a psychiatric hospital was $607, compared with $85 in prison, $64 in jail, and $38 in a public shelter.[49] What this comparison ignores, however, are the multiple social service, police, and court costs associated with repeated arrests and jailings of untreated mentally ill persons. It also ignores the human costs associated with homelessness, incarceration, and episodes of violence. If the proper laws and safeguards are in place and used, as discussed in chapter 11, the total cost of excellent treatment for individuals with severe psychiatric disorders is surprisingly close to the cost of providing no treatment at all. Whatever money is saved by failing to treat mentally ill persons comes at a very high price.

Lost Lives

In an attempt to fully understand the failure of psychiatric services in California, I wrote to Herb Mullin to request an interview. He wrote back granting permission and sent copies of his writings and appeals for parole. In September 2005, I visited him at Mule Creek State Prison, in Ione, where the Sacramento plain meets the Sierra foothills. From the prison, one can see the golden hills reaching upward toward Jackson and Sutter Creek, the heart of gold rush country.

In the prison visiting room, he greeted me briskly, formally. He is a small man with a receding hairline and looked older than his fifty-eight years; he seemed an unlikely candidate to have killed thirteen people. In our two-hour conversation, he willingly answered all my questions and was eager for me to understand that he is no longer sick and is anxious to get out of prison. He would like to get married, he said, and start a family. He assured me that he and his wife "would help each other and would be good citizens."

I asked him about his diagnosis of schizophrenia. Both in our conversation and in subsequent correspondence, he stated emphatically that he had healed himself: "I discarded the disease, left it behind me, somewhere in the past." He acknowledged that he did have schizophrenia at the time of the crimes but believes it had been caused by his family and friends. He was "naïve and gullible," he said, and claimed he had been subjected to "psychological sadism" and "psychologically forced to commit the crimes." Moreover, he believes that "during the four-month period they [his family and friends] knew when each one of the thirteen murders took place, yet they did nothing to notify the sheriff." It is they, not he, who should have been prosecuted, he believes. His schizophrenia, he claimed, was a "family-induced internal conflict," words he took directly from the writings of the English psychiatrist Ronald Laing, whom he regards as having had a correct understanding of the disease.

Herb Mullin is sincere in his beliefs about what happened and his own lack of personal responsibility for the crimes. He says he feels bad for the victims and prays for them. He also prays daily: "Eternal life. God bless America. Wealth and health. Improvement guaranteed." His parents are both deceased, and he has had no contact with his sister or any other relative or friend for many years. He prefers it that way, since he believes they were responsible for his problems. In relating these things, he did so without emotion, as if he were discussing what the prison serves for lunch. He has no more awareness of his illness now than he had thirty-five years ago.

According to officials at the prison, Mullin is a model prisoner. He keeps his cell immaculate, participates in activities, and causes no problems. He has not taken any psychiatric medication for almost twenty years and refuses to consider it, since he is certain that he is no longer sick. Mullin even wonders whether the Thorazine he was given during his first hospitalization might have caused his schizophrenia. According to California state law, prisoners cannot be forced to take psychiatric medication unless they are causing problems and are considered to be a danger to themselves or others, and only then by court order. The law completely protects Herb Mullin's civil rights, including his right to remain delusional for the rest of his life. At the end of our interview, I walked back through the steel doors and into the sunshine, profoundly depressed.

Herb Mullin is one of 162,000 persons in the California state prison system. Since 20 percent of them are, like Mullin, seriously mentally ill, that means that there are approximately 32,000 mentally ill prisoners. Coincidentally or not, that is the number of beds that were closed over the years in the state psychiatric hospitals. At $85 per day, Mullin's incarceration has so far cost California's taxpayers over one million dollars, and may well cost another one million before he dies.

And what about the lives lost? How do you put a price on those? Lawrence White, Fred Perez, and Father Tomei, given their ages, would probably have died from other causes by now. Mary Guilfoyle, Jim and Joan Gianera, Kathy Francis, David Oliker, Rob Spector, Scott Card, and Mark Dreibelbis would be in their fifties, while David and Daemon Francis would just be in their forties. The long-term effect of these deaths on their families and relatives can only be imagined. As Kenneth Springer, foreman of Mullin's jury, summarized it, "None of this need ever have happened."

The Legacy of the Lanterman-Petris-Short Act

The implementation of LPS in 1969 is the most important reason for the continuing failure in California to treat individuals with severe psychiatric disorders. This failure has been a major contributor to the following situations:

- It is estimated that at least 38,000 severely mentally ill individuals are homeless on any given day, the majority being in Los Angeles and San Francisco.
- Approximately 9,000 severely mentally ill individuals are in county jails, constituting 11 percent of all individuals in jails in California.
- Approximately 32,000 severely mentally ill individuals are in state prisons, constituting 20 percent of all state prisoners.
- Between 1970 and 2004, severely mentally ill individuals, most of whom were not receiving treatment, were responsible for at least 4,700 California homicides. Each year, they are responsible for an additional 120 homicides.

5 | The Killing of Three Devils

When the personal freedom of the mentally ill is given priority
over all other considerations, the tyranny of some will jeopardize
the autonomy of all.

GARY J. MAIER, M.D., 1989

The events of February 7, 1985, at St. Patrick's Catholic Church
stunned the western Wisconsin town of Onalaska. Mayor Van Riper
didn't believe it: "I thought, 'You've got to be kidding—those things don't
happen here.'"[1] Sandra Beitlich, a fifteen-year resident, added, "It's scary to
think it could happen in such a small town. . . . Church is supposed to be
a sacred place and to have something like this happen is just kind of sick."
That the priest had been praying at the altar when he was killed was rem-
iniscent of T. S. Eliot's *Murder in the Cathedral*.

Situated on bluffs overlooking the confluence of the Black, La
Crosse, and Mississippi Rivers, Onalaska seemed an unlikely setting for
such a crime. The town's most exciting event had traditionally been the
annual New Year's Eve fireworks. Its 15,000 residents, mostly of European immigrant stock, celebrated a Norwegian Folk Festival in the
summer, an Oktoberfest in the fall, and a Snowflake Ski Jumping Tour-
nament in the winter. Onalaska had once been a thriving lumber town,
but many of its residents now commuted to service jobs in La Crosse,

five miles to the south. The Native American name of the town meant "dwelling together harmoniously."

February 7 dawned clear and very cold. Few people had noticed twenty-nine-year-old Bryan Stanley as he walked along Main Street carrying a black gun case, his yellow Michelob stocking cap pulled down over his ears. Carrying a gun is relatively common in Wisconsin, which has more hunters per capita than any other state. Although Stanley had grown up in La Crosse, going to Catholic elementary school there and graduating from Central High School, he was at the time living in Onalaska and was known to many townspeople, including the local police.

St. Patrick's Catholic Church, which serves about eight hundred families, has a modern brick-and-wood interior; above the altar a large picture of Jesus looks down from the cross. Bryan Stanley knew the church well. His brother-in-law had taken him there in February 1983. At the time, Stanley was agitated and convinced that "the devil was tormenting him and playing tricks, like making street lights go out when he walked under them." He had also been standing in the middle of the street, "totally oblivious to cars," and later had "tried jumping out of the car going 40 mph." Stanley had calmed down somewhat when he got to the church, assured by his brother-in-law that "the devil can't get you in church."

Over the next two years, Bryan Stanley had returned periodically to St. Patrick's. On another occasion, while praying at the Catholic Cathedral in La Crosse, he had heard the Virgin Mary say, "St. Patrick would like you to go to Onalaska and pray at his church." He did so, sometimes "for hours at a time." Two weeks prior to the murders, Stanley had caused a disturbance at St. Patrick's; the police took him to a hospital in La Crosse for a psychiatric examination, and he was released. His behavior, however, was sufficiently threatening that the Onalaska Police Department was said to be keeping an eye on him. On February 4, at the La Crosse Catholic Cathedral, Stanley had announced to the priests there that he was the prophet Elijah. According to the account of one priest, "They thought he was harmless. . . . Churches become the havens for many types of people and you treat them gently; you don't call the police just because someone says he is a prophet."

On February 6, Stanley attended morning Mass at St. Patrick's. A Catholic elementary school was attached to the church, and children were allowed to read the day's lessons. On this particular morning, a girl read one of the lessons. In recent months, Stanley had complained many times that the Catholic Church had become too liberal and that only males should read the Scriptures. He was so upset that he left the Mass early. That night, Stanley saw a program on television about girls being allowed to take part in the Catholic Mass, and this left him further disturbed.

He awoke early on February 7, determined to get to St. Patrick's before the 8 a.m. Mass. The Virgin Mary had told him to ask the priest if he was going to again let a girl read the Scriptures. At a few minutes before eight, Stanley knocked on the door of the sacristy where Father John Rossiter was preparing for Mass. Carrol Pederson and Ferdinand Roth, both lay ministers, were with Rossiter. Stanley asked the priest whether he was going to allow a girl to read the Scriptures during Mass, and Rossiter acknowledged that he was. "That's not right," said Stanley. "Who said you could do that?" "The Pope told me I can do that, and that is good enough for me," replied Rossiter, shutting the door.

Bryan Stanley was furious. He went to a nearby restaurant, had some coffee, and tried to call the Catholic bishop in La Crosse. The line was busy. He looked at a morning newspaper—the print and pictures were standing out in three dimensions. Some of the pictures even looked like saints. Clearly, these were signs, like so many of the signs he had been receiving. The three men in the sacristy must be devils, and he had been sent as Elijah to purify the church. As he later recalled, "I had a duty to save the world from war, communism and sin. . . . It was me versus the devil and communism. . . . I thought the world was coming to an end." He understood his mission.

Bryan Stanley walked purposefully up Main Street, turned north on Second Avenue, and soon arrived at the small white house he shared with his childhood friend Cass Schrabeck. The back of the house over-

looks the Mississippi River, and in autumn the high bluffs on the Minnesota side of the river turn orange and yellow, a picture of northern
tranquillity. Once in the house, Stanley went to Cass's gun rack. Stanley
owned several guns himself, but they were at his parents' home in La
Crosse. He selected a Remington 12-gauge pump shotgun and noticed
that it held three shells. Here was yet another sign: he was the third-
born child in his family, his mother had been thirty-three when he was
born, and Christ had been thirty-three when he died. Stanley put a few
extra shells in his pocket, just in case.

Stanley arrived back at the church just before nine. The Mass had
finished a few minutes earlier, and the children had returned to their
classrooms across the courtyard. When Stanley entered the church, it was
empty except for Father Rossiter, who was praying at the altar, as he
routinely did after Mass.

Father Rossiter, at the age of sixty-four, had been at St. Patrick's for
more than two decades. A University of Wisconsin at Madison graduate and World War II veteran, he was extremely popular with his
parishioners and with the schoolchildren for his "keen Irish wit." He
was said to be "a joy to be around . . . all Irish in every way you can
possibly imagine. . . . He made everyone feel that they were the most
important person in the world." Bryan Stanley's family also knew and
admired Father Rossiter; he had even performed the marriage of one
of Bryan's sisters and baptized her two children.

Stanley took the gun out of its case and walked up the aisle to within
ten feet of the kneeling priest. At the last moment, Father Rossiter
turned. Stanley shot him in the face and then moved quickly toward
the door that led to the sacristy. Inside, fifty-five-year-old Ferdinand
Roth was preparing to join his wife, Nancy, who was waiting outside
in their van. Roth, a Korean War veteran, had worked as a lay minister
with Father Rossiter for eight years after a bad back forced him to
retire from the railroad. He had six children, and one of his grandsons
had been in the group of children he had been training that morning
to help serve Mass. Roth saw Stanley coming and tried to run but was
caught with a shot to the back of his neck.

That left one more. As Bryan Stanley later recalled, "I then had to find a third man. It could have been anybody." The voices had talked about "the three devils in the church. . . . I didn't even think of them as human. . . . They were all evil and talking amongst themselves." Stanley went to the basement, where he saw William Hammes, age sixty-five, a retired truck driver and World War II veteran who was the church janitor. His wife supervised the church school playground, and his daughter played the church organ for services. As Stanley described it, Hammes "went into a room and tried to close the door but I would not let him. He was lying on the floor and he knew what was going to happen to him. I shot him in the back of the head."

Bryan Stanley had done his job as "a soldier of Christ." He placed the gun in its case and started walking east on Main Street. Voices told him that there were also three devils at the Blessed Sacrament Church in La Crosse, so he had more work to do. He had gone only six blocks when he was spotted by Deputy Sheriff Randy Haller, who was responding to the 911 call from the church. Haller ordered Stanley to drop his gun, put up his hands, and identify himself. Stanley replied that his name was Elijah and that he needed to talk to the pope.

Waiting for the World to Stop

In the weeks that followed, the events leading up to the murders were examined, publicly and privately, in minute detail. As Onalaska Police Sergeant Bob Muth described it, "You just keep asking why. Were there things we could have done to stop this?" For Muth, it was also a personal loss; he had been working closely with Father Rossiter as he converted to Catholicism, and the two men had become close friends.

There was nothing in Bryan Stanley's early history that foreshadowed the tragedy. The third of seven children in a stable Catholic family, his father worked as a tool designer at a local factory. He had been "an average kid" with average grades and a member of the track team at La Cross Central High School. After graduation, he had started college at the University of Wisconsin at La Crosse but then switched to the Stevens Point campus in order to major in soil science. After receiving his degree in 1977, he went to work for the Federal Forest Service mapping soils in South Dakota and Wisconsin. He had a girlfriend and many male friends and appeared to be a normal young man embarking on a normal life course.

In 1981, at age twenty-six, he decided to join the Army to learn a language and do some traveling. He completed basic training without difficulty and was assigned to the language training school in Monterey, California. He found the class work extremely difficult and was reassigned three months later to be trained as an X-ray technician in Texas. There, he remembers feeling "spaced out all the time" and underwent counseling for depression and suicidal feelings. He was sent next to Walter Reed Army Hospital in Washington, D.C., for additional technician training, and he continued to receive psychotherapy.

In February 1983, Stanley was assigned to duty at an Army Reserve base in Pennsylvania. By this time, he had become preoccupied with the Bible. In response to verbal instructions from God, Stanley went AWOL and returned home. He called his family together and said he had good news. They expected he would announce his engagement, but instead he started reading from the Bible and preaching to them. His mother suspected he had been "brainwashed by a religious cult," especially the following day when he "came dashing out of his bedroom in his underwear, yelling that the devil was after him." Shortly thereafter, his brother-in-law took him to St. Patrick's Catholic Church, where, he said, the devil could not get him. He was hospitalized at St. Francis Hospital in La Crosse and diagnosed for the first time with schizophrenia.

Over the next two years, Bryan Stanley was psychiatrically hospitalized or evaluated at least seven times. After an inpatient stay of four months at Walter Reed Army Hospital, he was discharged from the Army with a disability pension of $590 per month. He was hospitalized for six weeks at Newberry State Hospital in Michigan after "he attacked his [job] supervisor because he thought he was the devil and he was hearing his supervisor's voice in his head." When a police officer tried to arrest him for this attack, Stanley attacked the arresting officer. Stanley had demonstrated his propensity for violence during his first hospitalization in La Crosse, when he "attacked a patient on the ward and began to choke her but was eventually restrained."

When Bryan Stanley was given antipsychotic medication during his hospitalizations, he responded rapidly. Each time he left the hospital, however, he stopped taking it, usually within a week, according to an analysis of medication bottles found among his belongings after the murders. Hospital staff noted that he did not take medication voluntarily, because he did not believe that he was sick or that anything was wrong with him. One psychiatrist who examined him summarized, "I believe that it has been clearly demonstrated many times in the past that Mr. Stanley does exceedingly well while on medications, but becomes quite psychotic and disorganized when not taking them."[2]

In the weeks leading up to the murders, Bryan Stanley had become increasingly psychotic. One night, God told him to "light a candle," so he walked downtown in the middle of the night looking for a candle. Police took him to St. Francis Hospital for evaluation, but he was released without treatment. Two days later, he was again picked up by the police. He was waiting for the "world to stop," he said, and identified himself as Christ. He was hospitalized overnight and released. His parents were extremely worried, but they knew little about mental illness and no one told them their son had schizophrenia. His mother called him "confused and tormented." His father later said he had assumed that the "hospitals would see that Bryan got the necessary treatment," but the hospitals kept releasing him without treatment. What was the family supposed to do?

The *Lessard* Decision

The main reason Bryan Stanley did not receive adequate treatment during the two years in which his psychosis deepened was that Wisconsin's mental health laws did not allow it. At that time in Wisconsin, the *involuntary* hospitalization and treatment of individuals like Bryan

Stanley was virtually impossible. The law stated that there must be proof "that there is an *extreme* likelihood that if the person is not confined he will do *immediate* harm to himself or other . . . and dangerousness is based upon a finding of a *recent* overt act, attempt or threat to do *substantial* harm to oneself or another" (emphasis added). Stanley's violent attacks on others had happened months before, so they did not qualify as "recent." He had gone for long periods in the community untreated, so how could one say the potential harm would be "immediate"? And what exactly was "extreme likelihood" or "substantial harm"? Believing that God was talking to you or that you were Elijah did not, by itself, qualify you as being dangerous.

The Wisconsin law, implemented in 1975, was a product of the *Lessard* decision issued by a U.S. District Court three years earlier. The law previous to *Lessard* had been much more liberal, allowing for involuntary hospitalization of an individual on the basis of "clear and convincing evidence" that the person was "mentally ill." This law was typical of commitment statutes in most states at that time.

The plaintiff had been Alberta Lessard, a forty-nine-year-old former schoolteacher who was living in West Allis, a suburb of Milwaukee. She had grown up in Ingram (population 153), in northern Wisconsin, where her father was a lumberjack and camp cook and her mother a self-taught midwife. Ms. Lessard had worked in restaurants to put herself through Eau Claire Teachers College, then got a master's degree in education at Marquette University and earned most of the credits required for a doctorate. Her twenty-six-year teaching career had included stints in primary schools in Rusk, Chippewa, Marathon, and Washington Counties before she ended up in West Allis. In 1967, at age forty-five, she had been fired by the school board because of her behavior, which apparently concerned her failure to follow specified teaching practices.

For the next four years, Alberta Lessard experienced increasing difficulties with her neighbors and with local authorities. This friction culminated on October 29, 1971, when police were called to her apartment house three separate times. According to the police report, Ms.

Lessard was "running up and down the apartment aisle on the second floor banging on doors and shouting that the communists were taking over the country that night." According to one of the officers, Ms. Lessard "kept saying over and over that the communists were taking over . . . and that we should do something right away. She kept talking about burning some evidence in her sink, evidence of her as a bubble dancer . . . some caricature or picture depicting her as a bubble dancer. She said she had burned this along with other evidence, something to do with a secret invention." She was also alleged to have jumped from her second-story window and "said that she no longer had the will to live and that she might, if returned to the apartment, jump again."[3] The police officers took Ms. Lessard to the Milwaukee Mental Health Center, where she was involuntarily committed for being mentally ill.

A preliminary psychiatric evaluation found that Ms. Lessard was suffering from paranoid schizophrenia and was in need of treatment. She retained counsel through the Milwaukee Legal Services, a federal- and state-funded organization that provided legal assistance for low-income individuals. Robert Blondis and Thomas Dixon, two young lawyers who had recently completed their training, took the case. Rather than defend only Ms. Lessard, they decided instead to file a class action suit on behalf of "all other persons 18 years of age and older who are being held involuntarily pursuant to any emergency, temporary or permanent commitment provision of the Wisconsin involuntary commitment statute." For activist young lawyers like Blondis and Dixon, filing a class action was consistent with the civil rights milieu of that era. In a later interview, Blondis frankly admitted that, at the time, he "knew nothing about mental health law," adding, "I had read a few things, including Thomas Szasz's *The Myth of Mental Illness*, and that is where I was coming from." Szasz's 1961 book explicitly denied that mental illness exists in any scientific sense but was instead merely arbitrarily defined categories of behavior. In researching their class action suit, Blondis recalled "sitting around one evening in the basement law library drinking beer," when they came across the phrase "least restrictive alternative" in a totally unrelated legal case involving state employees in Arkansas. They inserted the phrase into their class action suit, and it subsequently became widely used to justify the release of psychiatric patients from hospitals.[4]

In October 1972, one year after the class action suit had been filed, a three-judge panel of the U.S. District Court declared Wisconsin's existing civil commitment statute unconstitutional. It said that proof of mental illness and dangerousness must be proven "beyond a reasonable doubt," a much more rigorous legal standard than the existing "clear and convincing evidence." Involuntary hospitalization should be used "only as a last resort" when there are not "less drastic means for achieving the same basic goal." The *Lessard* decision was called "the first landmark case dealing with the concept of dangerousness . . . a high-water mark in 'dangerousness' law."[5]

The *Lessard* decision was strongly influenced by the theories of the psychiatrist Thomas Szasz, just as the Lanterman-Petris-Short Act in California had been five years earlier. In their decision, the three judges noted, "Obviously, the definition of mental illness is left largely to the user and is dependent upon the norms of adjustment that he employs. . . . The diagnostician has the ability to shoehorn into the mentally diseased class almost any person he wishes, for whatever reason, to put there." In addition to Szasz, the other eminence grise behind the *Lessard* decision was Bruce Ennis, then director of the Mental Illness Litigation Project for the New York Civil Liberties Union. Ennis had also been strongly influenced by Szasz and, as noted in chapter 1, had dedicated himself to "nothing less than the abolition of involuntary hospitalization." In 1969, in testimony before a U.S. Senate subcommittee, Ennis had recommended, "Commitment because of alleged danger to self or to others should require proof beyond a reasonable doubt, based on a recent overt act or threat, that the person would, if at liberty, inflict substantial physical injury upon himself or others within the immediate future."[6] The *Lessard* decision included exactly the same wording: "beyond a reasonable doubt" as its standard of proof and "a recent overt act," "substantial harm to oneself or another," and "immediate harm" as its standards of dangerousness.

The influence of both Szasz and Ennis was also seen in perhaps the most important aspect of the *Lessard* decision. In his 1969 Senate testimony, Ennis had said, "A patient suffering from cancer, heart disease, or pneumonia can't be committed, even for his own welfare. Apparently, involuntary treatment of the mental patient is based on the assumption first, that he is incompetent to make a 'rational' choice between liberty and treatment, and second, that he would, if competent, choose treatment. There is not to my knowledge any evidence to support either of these assumptions." Szasz had similarly claimed that "the argument that so-called mentally ill persons do not know what they 'really' need for their own welfare is deceptive." The *Lessard* judges mirrored such thinking when writing their decision: "Persons in need of hospitalization for mental illness should be allowed choice of whether to undergo hospitalization and treatment or not unless the state can prove that the person is unable to make decisions about hospitalization because of [the] nature of illness."[7] The court did not further define what it meant by "unable to make decisions" or how the state was supposed to establish this deficit.

The practical effect of Wisconsin's 1975 law passed in the wake of *Lessard*, as noted one year later by the legal scholar Alan Stone, was to "put a virtual end to involuntary confinement" of psychiatric patients if the law was strictly followed. This was, of course, exactly what the framers of the law intended. The Wisconsin psychiatrist Darold Treffert similarly observed, "Provisions for the state to use *parens patriae* [protection of people who cannot protect themselves] powers in the absence of dangerousness narrowly defined were effectively abolished; the pendulum swung entirely to dangerousness in terms of imminent physical harm as the only authority on which the state could infringe on individual liberty."[8]

"Four Wasted Lives"

The trial of Bryan Stanley in October 1985 was a national event. ABC, CBS, *USA Today*, and the Associated Press sent reporters. Minneapolis television crews came by helicopter and truck. The trial was carried live on three cable stations and the radio, and media inquiries were received from Britain, France, and Australia—the La Crosse County Courthouse had never seen anything like it.

Stanley had not elicited much sympathy from the public. At his initial hearing, he had "yelled obscenities and talked for 15 minutes about being a 'soldier for Christ.'" He also telephoned a reporter and told him that he had "killed for Christ": "I meant to kill them. I'm not crazy. The public thinks I am crazy but I am not. I had a job to do and I did it well."

By contrast, there was an outpouring of sympathy for the victims' families. At a joint funeral service in the La Crosse Catholic Cathedral, over two thousand mourners "packed the cathedral, filing in hours before the service" and overflowing to the basement, where many watched the service on television. Father Bernard McGarty, a close personal friend of Father Rossiter, told those assembled that "the Lord does not will evil but He does permit evil [as] the price we pay for the possibility of freedom."

After being charged with three counts of murder, Bryan Stanley was transferred to Mendota Mental Health Institute in Madison for psychiatric evaluation. He was given antipsychotic medication, and, as before, the symptoms of his schizophrenia rapidly abated. In less than three months, he was said to have "improved dramatically" and to "no longer believe God ordered him to kill three people."

When he went to trial in October, Bryan Stanley was completely free of psychotic symptoms. Multiple psychiatrists had examined him in the intervening months; all agreed that he had schizophrenia and that he had been psychotic at the time of the murders. With the agreement of both the prosecution and the defense, his three-day trial was held before a judge only. Stanley acknowledged that he had killed the men but pleaded not guilty by reason of mental disease.

The outcome of the trial surprised no one. The judge ruled that Stanley had been insane at the time of the murders and was not legally responsible because he "lacked substantial capacity to appreciate the wrongfulness of his actions and to conform his conduct to the requirements of the law." In his ruling, the judge questioned the competence of the La Crosse hospital personnel who had evaluated Stanley twice shortly before the murders but had failed to treat him. On the day of the ruling, Mary Stanley, Bryan's mother, publicly asserted that if her son "had been forced to take his medication, he might not have killed anyone. . . . This whole thing is such a tragedy, there was just four wasted lives."

6 | The Sad Legacy of Ms. Lessard

The "freedom" to be penniless, helpless, ill, and finally arrested, jailed and criminally committed is not freedom at all—it is abandonment. . . . The "liberty" to be naked in a padded cell, hallucinating, delusional, and tormented, is not liberty—it is a folie à deux *between pseudo-sophisticated liberals and an unrealizing public.*

DAROLD TREFFERT, 1982

By the time Bryan Stanley killed three people in February 1985, it had become cruelly clear that the 1972 *Lessard* decision had precipitated a human disaster. The three-judge panel had essentially reversed seven hundred years of English civil law that established government's responsibility to protect individuals who are unable to protect themselves, the principle of *parens patriae*. The Wisconsin law ignored *parens patriae* and assumed that mentally ill individuals were competent to decide whether they needed treatment. The new law established extremely strict criteria for dangerousness and made them the only grounds for involuntary treatment. As a legal scholar summarized shortly after the *Lessard* decision was handed down, "the decision effectively obliterated a major portion of the Wisconsin civil commitment statute."[1]

The use of narrowly defined dangerousness as the sole criterion for involuntary treatment produced judicial absurdities that became manifest immediately following the implementation of the *Lessard* ruling. For example:

- A young woman with schizophrenia was evicted from a group home for setting fires. At her parents' house, "she began to use words like kill," and her parents "would wake up in the middle of the night and she'd be in our bedroom standing over us." After the daughter assaulted her mother, the mother applied for an involuntary commitment. "She was told that even though her daughter had struck her, she hadn't been hit hard enough." "They asked me if I had bruises," she said.
- A young man with schizophrenia "claimed he was dead" and stored his urine in bottles under his bed. He said that his mother was not his real mother and "threatened to cut her into pieces." According to a newspaper account, when the mother petitioned for involuntary commitment, the judge denied it: "The man merely had threatened to cut his mother with a knife, the judge noted. There was no evidence introduced that he ever actually chased her around the house with one."
- A young woman with schizophrenia had "once set fire to a bathroom to get rid of demons" and "threw a chair and began beating it against the partition in a social worker's office." When the woman "began walking around the streets naked," her mother petitioned for involuntary commitment. The judge denied it, saying that "there was not enough evidence of dangerousness as defined by state law."[2]

An especially egregious example of the consequences of the *Lessard* decision occurred in Milwaukee in October 1980. A man with schizophrenia was jailed "for making sexual comments to people on a bus." While in jail, he refused food but was observed eating his feces. He was therefore transferred to a psychiatric hospital for evaluation, and a petition was filed requesting involuntary psychiatric commitment and treatment. Robert Gregor, a psychiatrist, testified that the man was mentally ill and in need of treatment. Attorney Stuart Spielman, a pub-

lic defender, argued that the man did not meet the standard of dangerousness required under Wisconsin laws:

Atty. Spielman: "Isn't it correct that he has been eating meals at the hos-
   pital?"
Dr. Gregor: "He just started to eat a day or two ago."
Atty. Spielman: "Doctor, at present, he is in no imminent physical peril,
   is that correct?"
Dr. Gregor: "Apparently not, since he started to eat."
Atty. Spielman: "Would the eating of fecal material on one occasion by
   an individual pose a serious risk of harm to that person?"
Dr. Gregor: "It is certainly not edible material. . . . It contains elements
   that are certainly considered harmful or unnecessary."
Atty. Spielman: "But, doctor, you cannot state whether the consumption
   of such material on one occasion would invariably harm a person?"
Dr. Gregor: "Certainly not on one occasion."

Spielman then moved to dismiss the petition on the grounds that the
man was in no danger of physical injury or of dying. The judge agreed
and said the man did not qualify for involuntary commitment. In a
statement to the newspaper, Thomas Zander, another public defender,
supported the judge's decision, saying that the man had "behaved the
way he did to get attention" and that "he made a choice" to remain in
jail rather than go to the psychiatric hospital.

Once released from jail, the man was rearrested three times within
three months; following the third arrest, a different judge committed
him to a psychiatric hospital, where he was involuntarily treated.
"Within two or three days he began verbally requesting the medicine"
and "over the course of time he became fairly normal."[3]

"The New Lepers"

The magnitude of the disaster engendered by the revised commitment
statutes varied from county to county. According to a 1976 study,

"many county judges disagreed with much of the *Lessard* decision" and initially interpreted the law more loosely. Over time, however, it became increasingly difficult to get a mentally ill person committed for treatment anywhere in the state. In Milwaukee, for example, approximately one out of every two petitions for commitment had been approved in 1974, prior to implementation of the new laws. By 1983, the approval rate decreased to one in twelve, and by 1995, to one in fifty. Newspapers carried accounts of "dozens and dozens of families each year who are desperately trying to get help for their loved ones but can't because the law won't let them."[4] Bryan Stanley was merely one of thousands of severely mentally ill individuals in Wisconsin who did not receive needed psychiatric treatment in the years following the *Lessard* decision.

The failure to treat these persons spurred an increase in the number of mentally ill who became homeless. In Milwaukee, this was said to be "a new concern" in 1980, but by 1982 stories such as "Number of Homeless Is Straining Shelters" were being regularly reported. By 1984, a headline read, "Homeless Mentally Ill: Problem Is Growing, Showing"; it was said to be "one of the city's most visible social problems" and led to a conference with "200 mental health and social service officials." In 1986, a formal survey of homeless individuals found that "27 percent have been hospitalized for mental problems." With each passing year, the number of mentally ill homeless increased; by 2000, it was estimated "that half of the 2,000 or so who live on Milwaukee's streets are chronically and persistently mentally ill."[5]

Vance Baker, a psychiatrist who worked with Milwaukee's homeless population, said, "The legal system is an impediment to the treatment of many of these people." They therefore continued to live on the streets, increasing in numbers each year:

- John, from a middle-class suburban Milwaukee home, sleeps under a footbridge, hears God whispering to him, feels "silverfish crawling all over his body," and eats "garbage out of the trash cans in the alleys of the east side."
- Virgie, in her mid-fifties, "carries a plastic doll and wears a long coat

over a see-through nightie." In the bus depot, she "opens up her coat" and "parades around like a fashion model."

- A man known to the police as "the mechanic" carries a tool box and periodically goes into commercial establishments and tries to repair machines. "He once walked into a McDonald's restaurant restroom and removed the toilet and the towel cabinet."
- Betty, sitting next to the post office with her shopping bags, has been raped nine times.

A nun who worked with Milwaukee's mentally ill called them "the new lepers—people want to tuck them into a corner and forget about them."[6]

The best-known mentally ill homeless person in Milwaukee was the late Lionel Aldridge, a former all-pro linebacker for Wisconsin's beloved Green Bay Packers. After retiring from football, he developed paranoid schizophrenia and was homeless on Milwaukee's streets for several years. When he took medication, which he did intermittently, he was a public spokesperson for mentally ill persons. However, when he did not take it, he was psychotic and homeless like so many others. Even though he was an esteemed Green Bay Packer, Wisconsin's laws made it impossible to treat Lionel Aldridge involuntarily.[7]

"Human Beings Rotting Away"

Darold Treffert started talking about the "balloon theory" as soon as Wisconsin's new commitment laws went into effect. The theory, originally expounded by Lionel Penrose in 1939, posits that the populations of psychiatric hospitals and prisons are inversely correlated—as one decreases, the other increases.[8] Push in on one side of the balloon, and the other side will bulge out.

Treffert was well placed to observe these effects. When the *Lessard* decision was handed down, he was the thirty-eight-year-old director of Winnebago State Hospital, one of the state's three psychiatric hospitals. After the new laws were implemented, Treffert noticed an increase in the number of mentally ill patients admitted to his hospital who also had been arrested or who had existing criminal charges. Treffert was one of the first psychiatrists in the United States to chronicle this emerging national trend, and he published his observations in an article entitled "Legal 'Rites': Criminalizing the Mentally Ill."[9] Treffert, who was also president of both the Wisconsin Psychiatric Association and the Wisconsin Medical Society, became the state's leading critic of the *Lessard* decision.

By 1981, the criminalization of mentally ill persons in Wisconsin had become obvious and was being documented by the media. A survey of jails done at the time estimated that "about 13 percent of the inmates were diagnosed as having mental disabilities." The *Milwaukee Sentinel* published a series of exposés, noting that "mentally ill people are turning up in Wisconsin's prisons and jails at an alarming rate. . . . Sheriffs and prison administrators are grimly aware of the situation and have reported significant increases in the number of prisoners who apparently need mental health care rather than a prison cell." At the Milwaukee County Jail:

- A woman with "a long history of mental illness" died naked on the concrete floor of her cell. She had been arrested for exposing herself on the street.
- A sixty-four-year-old man was placed in solitary confinement "because he urinated and defecated on himself, sometimes eating his own feces. Deputies had to throw buckets of strong detergent into his cell . . . several times each day to defeat the smell."[10]

In Wisconsin's state prisons, the situation was even worse. According to one report, "the state's prison population tripled in the decade beginning in 1980, largely with prisoners who were mentally ill and in the past would have been in mental hospitals." At the Waupun State Prison, a newspaper described a young man with schizophrenia sitting "naked in his own excrement . . . exhibiting masturbatory behavior." Although the man had been successfully treated with antipsychotic medication in the past, after the new mental health laws were passed and those treating him had to abide by his refusal of medication, it was said that "when he talks, it's usually an odd, irrational phrase." Richard Arnesen, the prison's psychiatrist, was quoted as saying, "I've seen this man deteriorate little by little . . . to the point where he is hardly more than a vegetable. . . . These are human beings rotting away, getting worse and worse and worse."[11]

Reports described life for mentally ill prisoners in Wisconsin's jails and prisons as atrocious, with suicides on the increase. The director of the State Division of Corrections noted, "It's probably the cruelest kind of situation . . . to have a mentally ill person in a large prison where there is a great deal of impersonalization. Predators are always present." Mentally ill prisoners were said to be "vulnerable to sexual attacks, beatings, verbal harassment and thefts." Other inmates did not want to share a cell, or even a cellblock, with them. One prisoner acknowledged having beaten up his new, mentally ill cellmate as "the only way to get rid of him." Another prisoner wrote, "Do you think that you could stomach walking past a prisoner's cell and look in, and there he sits in the middle of the floor rubbing excrement up and down his arm, all over his beard and all up and down his legs?" Waupun prison's chief psychologist described the situation as "something out of the Middle Ages" but said that the laws made involuntary treatment virtually impossible: "There's nothing to be done. They simply rot. They sit and rot."[12]

In the quarter century since these newspaper exposés were published, the situation for mentally ill individuals in Wisconsin's jails and prisons has continued to deteriorate. In 2000, it was estimated that "chronically mentally ill" individuals constituted 7 percent of the jail population, 15 to 20 percent of the prison population, and 20 percent of the people on parole or probation—a total of approximately 17,000 individuals. Among all state prison inmates in solitary confinement, called segregation units, it was said that 42 percent were "severely and persistently mentally ill." As one corrections officer explained, "the seg unit is literally a loony bin." In recent years, these numbers have continued to climb; between 1999 and 2003, the costs for psychiatric medications in the Wisconsin prison system more than tripled.[13]

Although the criminalization of the mentally ill is most severe in

Milwaukee, it has occurred throughout the state. In La Crosse County in 2001, it was estimated that 7 to 10 percent of jail inmates had schizophrenia, bipolar disorder, or major depression; "we do seem to be getting more people with mental health needs," said the acting jail administrator. Most of the county's mentally ill inmates were not receiving treatment, a situation called "incomprehensibly inhumane" by La Crosse's mayor. Even in rural counties such as Trempealeau, the county jail was filled to capacity, and inmates were said to have "more serious medical and mental health complications."[14]

The progressive increase in mentally ill individuals in Wisconsin's jails and prisons had an obvious explanation—the *Lessard* decision and its consequent laws had practically guaranteed that they would not receive treatment for their mental illnesses. Untreated mentally ill individuals commit various misdemeanor and felony acts, usually related to their illness, and are thus arrested. In Milwaukee in 2000, it was said that "three dozen mentally ill people" were being arrested each day and that such cases constituted "40 percent of all those charged with disorderly conduct."[15]

Milwaukee police officers, after picking up mentally ill individuals who had committed misdemeanor crimes, initially took them to the county mental health facility for treatment. The usual outcome was described in 2000 by a police officer: "We take them out to the County Mental Health Complex to get them some help, only to be turned away. They say they've got no room. Often, we have no choice but to arrest them."[16] After a few such unsuccessful tries, most police officers gave up and instead took mentally ill persons directly to jail.

Police officers and jail personnel are not mental health professionals, and being forced into that role makes their job more difficult. In Wisconsin and elsewhere, corrections officers are now the front-line public officials who do most of the initial screening of mentally ill individuals. For trained mental health professionals, evaluating acutely psychotic individuals is a difficult job. For police officers with little or no training, it is an impossible task. "These are very volatile people," said one Milwaukee police officer; "we don't know what they will do from one minute to the next."[17]

Criminalizing the mentally ill also has economic consequences. In Wisconsin, as in California, state officials justified the closing of state hospital beds by saying that it saved money. In Milwaukee in 2000, a day in the county jail cost $60, a day in the state prison cost $200, and a day in the Milwaukee County Mental Health Complex cost $527. Shunting mentally ill individuals from psychiatric facilities to correctional facilities appears to save money overall, but these savings are largely illusory. They fail to account for the costs of repeated incarcerations, court proceedings, or the crimes committed. They also do not take into account the potential costs of civil judgments. In 1999, a federal jury awarded $5.4 million in compensatory and punitive damages to a Wisconsin man with schizophrenia who was incarcerated but not treated in the Monroe County Jail; it was said to be "the largest damage award to a person with a mental illness for lack of mental health treatment in jail."[18]

"Dying with One's Rights On"

In addition to accurately predicting the criminalization of mentally ill persons, Darold Treffert foresaw that the *Lessard* decision would have other untoward consequences. In the months after it was handed down, he began collecting examples of tragedies that appeared related to the new laws. He called these cases "dying with one's rights on" and published examples of them as early as 1973:

- A nineteen-year-old college student with schizoaffective disorder was hospitalized following a serious suicide attempt. Her family inquired about taking out commitment papers to ensure continued hospitalization but was told that their daughter did not meet commitment criteria under the new state laws, because she had not exhibited "extreme likelihood of immediate harm." The young woman signed herself out of the hospital and the following day hung herself.

- A forty-nine-year-old woman with severe anorexia admitted herself to a hospital but then insisted on signing out. The woman refused psychiatric help, so her family requested that she be involuntarily hospitalized to protect her. The judge ruled that the woman did not meet the new commitment criteria and released her. Three weeks later she starved to death.

Within a few years, Treffert cataloged over two hundred examples.[19]

Since Treffert's publication of these initial cases, *Lessard*-associated tragedies in Wisconsin have, like a steadily rising river, swept away more people each year. The tragedies include cases like those outlined above, but they also include individuals who are seriously injured or die in episodes of violence, or who kill others. It is this last group that the media are most likely to report on, and many of these cases have common components.

Family members are the most frequent targets when someone with an untreated psychiatric disorder becomes violent.

- **2000, Chippewa County:** Bill Marquardt, diagnosed with schizophrenia, killed his mother by stabbing her, and then shooting her in the head.
- **2004, Rock County:** Andrew Lubeck, diagnosed with bipolar disorder, killed his grandmother with a hammer because "she refused to write him a check."[20]

Incidents frequently involve police officers, who form the de facto front line in dealing with the mentally ill.

- **2004, Milwaukee:** Michael Blucher, diagnosed with schizophrenia, was killed by police after he moved toward them brandishing two large knives in an apparent "suicide by cop."
- **2005, Milwaukee:** Tou Yang, who believed that "the government was out to get him and that teachers were poisoning his children," was killed by police in a shootout.[21]

Many violent episodes involving individuals with severe psychiatric disorders are characterized by bizarre behavior consistent with the delusional thought patterns of those affected.

- **1998, Dunn County:** Kenneth Kartman pleaded not guilty by reason of insanity to a charge of attacking his father with a hatchet. He "had told his father that he would have to kill his family to prove that the hypothesis in the master's thesis on which he was working was correct."
- **1999, Racine County:** A fifty-one-year-old man diagnosed with bipolar disorder drove his car through a barricade and went airborne, "flying over another motorist" traveling on Highway 60 before crashing. The man told police he thought he had hit a speed bump.[22]

Mental health officials knew many of the perpetrators at the time of the tragedies. Some of them had been recently released from psychiatric hospitals.

- **1997, Pierce County:** Chad Blodgett, suffering from paranoid delusions, killed his two brothers "hours after he checked himself out of a psychiatric unit at a local hospital."
- **2001, Milwaukee:** A fifty-four-year-old woman started a fire in an apartment building, injuring five people; she had been taken into custody "10 times in the last 15 years for mental observations."[23]

The single most salient feature of these encounters is that almost all the mentally ill individuals were not taking medication at the time they occurred.

- **1991, Milwaukee:** Reginald Humphrey, diagnosed with paranoid schizophrenia but not taking his medication, "threw a gallon of gasoline at a woman in the University of Wisconsin–Milwaukee Student Union, then chased her through the building, throwing matches at her as she fled."

- **2004, Brown County:** Matthew Bradley, diagnosed with bipolar disorder but not taking his medication, bludgeoned his father to death with a hammer.[24]

The absence of any official registry that records tragedies like those listed above makes it impossible to quantify them with precision. Episodes in which mentally ill individuals are victimized or die because of the lack of adequate treatment are not kept in official statistics and are rarely reported by the media. Homicides by mentally ill individuals, however, are often reported, especially if the circumstances of the homicides are very strange or a prominent family is involved.

Despite the lack of precise numbers, it is apparent from a review of the news clippings maintained by the Treatment Advocacy Center that the incidence of tragedies involving individuals with severe psychiatric disorders has increased significantly in Wisconsin since the *Lessard* decision. The murders committed by Bryan Stanley in 1985 were merely the most highly publicized example, but such tragedies have continued to occur with disturbing regularity. The following episodes, for example, were reported by the Wisconsin media during a single eight-month period in 2003:

- **Trempealeau County:** Michael Crispin, diagnosed with schizophrenia but not taking his medication, was shot and killed by police after threatening them with a knife.
- **Milwaukee:** Lamarr Nash, diagnosed with schizophrenia and not taking his medication, led sheriff's deputies on a high-speed freeway chase broadcast on live television.
- **Waukesha County:** Brian Graf, diagnosed with paranoid schizophrenia, was arrested for assaulting a police officer.
- **Clark County:** Vernon Dukart, diagnosed with paranoid schizophrenia and not taking his medication, beat two neighbors with a hammer, killing one.
- **Winnebago County:** Gary Hirte pled not guilty by reason of insanity in the killing of a male friend.
- **Milwaukee:** Keith Addy, diagnosed with paranoid schizophrenia,

killed and dismembered the body of a woman who had come to his apartment from an escort service.

- **Dane County:** Roger O'Neal, diagnosed with paranoid schizophrenia, killed two of his stepsons and tried to kill another.
- **Walworth County:** Corey Dykas, diagnosed with schizophrenia, killed his parents because "voices in his head told him" to do so.
- **Sheboygan County:** Jason Larson, diagnosed with schizophrenia, killed his father and then shot at neighbors and the police. Two months earlier, Larson had "attempted to castrate himself."[25]

The "Madison Model" Mystery

Dane County, Wisconsin, which includes the city of Madison, is the third-wealthiest county in the state and has been reputed to have the best public psychiatric services in the United States. The "Madison model," considered to be the state of the art in American public psychiatry, has been lauded by the National Institute of Mental Health, the National Alliance for the Mentally Ill (which in 2005 changed its name to NAMI), and the National Association of Counties. It is used as a model for psychiatric services in thirty-three other states.

The "Madison model" is officially called the Program of Assertive Community Treatment, or PACT. It was developed by Leonard Stein and Mary Ann Test at the University of Wisconsin as a way to transition psychiatric patients from Mendota Mental Health Institute, located in Madison, to the community. PACT teams consist of five to fifteen mental health professionals who take full responsibility for groups of 100 to 200 psychiatric patients, twenty-four hours a day, seven days a week. PACT staff oversee not only the patients' medication maintenance but also their housing, vocational training, and rehabilitation. In contrast to traditional psychiatric services, in which professionals sit in their offices and let patients come to them, PACT staff spend the majority of their time in the community, meeting with patients wherever they are. One member of a PACT team is always on call to respond to crises.

The PACT model, when fully implemented, is highly effective. Studies have shown that for individuals with severe psychiatric disorders it can increase medication compliance, decrease hospitalizations, increase independent living, increase vocational success, decrease substance abuse, decrease time spent homeless, and decrease time spent in jail. Multiple economic analyses of the PACT model have shown that it costs no more than traditional models of psychiatric services when all costs, including law enforcement expenses and family burden, are taken into consideration.[26]

PACT was first put into operation in Dane County in 1972, coincidentally the same year in which the *Lessard* decision was handed down. Given the availability of a model program to deliver mental health services, one might expect that the untoward effects of the *Lessard* decision, such as homelessness, incarceration, victimization, and violence, would be less prevalent in Dane County than in other parts of Wisconsin. In fact, they are not.

Increased homelessness among mentally ill individuals was noted in Madison in the early 1980s. A citizens' organization representing several Madison churches carried out a study in 1982 and reported that "what we found was shocking." By 1984, one homeless shelter claimed that "half the population [using the shelter] is chronically mentally ill," and the following year a local newspaper claimed that "their numbers are growing in the wake of massive deinstitutionalization of the mentally troubled." By 1988, the *Capital Times* ran a three-part series on the problem of homelessness and estimated that the city had between 100 and 150 homeless persons in overflowing shelters and sleeping on the streets each night.[27]

The incarceration of mentally ill persons also became prominent in Dane County around this time. A 1984 study of young adults with schizophrenia in Madison found that 41 percent of them had been arrested at least once. A 1985 study reported that, during a four-month period, "59 persons were jailed for primarily psychiatric reasons," making the jail "a dumping ground for people who don't belong there." Madison newspapers described individuals such as a man, charged with disorderly conduct, "who goes by the alias Jesus Christ," and another "extremely psychotic" man, charged with "lewd and lascivious behavior," who "has been in jail 58 times charged with various misdemeanors." The reason for the criminalization of mentally ill individuals, according to the newspaper, was the *Lessard* decision, which made it "harder to commit people against their will" unless they were "immediately dangerous." Indeed, "even if mental health officials know that without treatment this person will become dangerous in a week or two, they cannot use the information to commit him."[28]

In 1988, at the same time that homelessness and the incarceration of mentally ill persons were increasing, it became dramatically evident that episodes of violence were also on the rise. Despite the "Madison model," Dane County, with a population of 350,000, in an eleven-month period experienced "six separate incidents [that] resulted in four homicides, three suicides, seven victims wounded by gunshot, and one victim mauled by a polar bear." Most prominent was the midday murder of the Dane County coroner, Clyde Chamberlain, and a secretary in Madison's City-County Building. The assailant, Aaron Lindh, was said to be "a little weird" and was well known to police for recent episodes of threatening people with guns. The county executive called the murders "the ultimate act of insanity."[29]

Less than two months after these homicides, a twenty-eight-year-old man climbed into the enclosure of Chief, a polar bear at the Madison Zoo. The man, who was said to have "been detained several times this year because of unstable actions" and had had two recent psychiatric hospital admissions, said he did so "to give his brother strength" and "to show courage." A police officer shot the bear, which was mauling the man, to save the man's life. According to the newspaper, the bear's death was said to be "the most eagerly discussed news story in Madison in weeks. . . . Many offered the opinion that [the police officer] should have shot the 28-year-old man instead of Chief," while others said the officer "should have walked away and let the bear kill the man." So strong was public opinion against the man that the *Capital Times* felt it necessary to run two editorials during the next week saying that "some people in Madison seem to have lost a sense of perspective." Meanwhile, a fund to purchase a new polar bear quickly raised over $50,000 in donations.[30]

The public sentiment favoring the bear over the man was a remarkable measure of how some people in Madison, a traditionally liberal community, had come to view mentally ill persons. The city's homeless shelters were overflowing, partly because of the number of mentally ill persons, and bitter disputes were occurring between neighborhoods trying to avoid becoming the site of a new shelter. The county jail was overcrowded; the director said his biggest frustration was "the high return rate of mentally ill people who are arrested for misdemeanors. . . . [O]ne man was arrested for such crimes as disorderly conduct and petty theft seven times in January."[31] Proposals for a new jail were under discussion despite the fact that already almost half of county property taxes were going to pay for the criminal justice system. Madison was said to have the best public psychiatric care system in the nation, yet by all visible measures it appeared to be a psychiatric disaster. What was going on?

In retrospect, the explanations are obvious. The highly praised PACT program in Dane County was, and is, available only to 140 severely mentally ill individuals, approximately 10 percent of the estimated total of 1,400 such individuals in need of such services. For that group of patients, PACT does an excellent job, with a consequent high level of medication compliance and a low level of homelessness and incarceration. For the rest of the county's severely mentally ill individuals, however, psychiatric services are deficient. An additional 30 percent of individuals with severe psychiatric disorders are served by four Community Support Programs (CSPs), which claim to be based on the PACT model but in reality are little more than traditional outpatient services. In 2006, the waiting list to receive either PACT or CSP services was two years long. An additional 25 percent of individuals with severe psychiatric disorders have only intermittent contact with the mental health system and may or may not be taking medication. The remaining 35 percent, including many of the homeless and the sickest individuals, are receiving no psychiatric care at all.

Dane County psychiatric services also are constrained by "a subtle antihospital bias" and a reluctance to employ involuntary treatment, even for patients who need it. A 1996 publication by Ronald Diamond, one of the county's leading psychiatrists, echoed these attitudes in praising the "continuing decrease in mental health commitments over the past ten years" and added, "Given the problems inherent in coercion, it would seem important to do everything possible to decrease the need for court-ordered treatment." Local mental health professionals are aware that their PACT program has been widely praised and appear to view involuntary treatment as a failure, even though PACT covers only about 10 percent of those who need it. In addition, Madison has the ambience of a liberal university town in which the word "involuntary" is considered an expletive. As described by Gary Maier, another Madison psychiatrist, psychiatry there "evolved over the years into an ideology . . . therapeutics turned into politics."[32]

Compounding Madison's problems at the time of the 1988 tragedies, and continuing to the present, has been a legal and judicial system also strongly biased against psychiatric hospitalization and involuntary treatment. Stuart Schwartz, a Dane County judicial court commissioner, represented this legal view. In 1985, he expressed doubt regarding the scientific validity of mental illness in general:

> *"You can see a broken leg," he says. "I'm still waiting for one of these doctors to describe to me . . . what a broken mind looks like. I'm waiting to find out: Is mental illness green? Can we cut it out?"*

In response to the increasing issues in Madison, Schwartz said that problems with the mentally ill in the community were perhaps "the price you have to pay in democracy."[33]

Dianne Greenley is another prominent Madison attorney who has zealously fought against all forms of involuntary treatment. Her response to the 1988 tragedies, which she called "extremely unfortunate incidents," was to observe that "violent actions by persons with mental illness are not always predictable." Greenley has unceasingly advocated for "patient rights" and "the elimination of involuntary commitment and other forced treatment." Regarding such advocacy efforts, Gary Maier observed, "I support the inalienable rights of patients, but I also support the inalienable responsibilities of patients. In their legalistic enthusiasm, advocates of strengthened patient rights have not kept the playing field balanced by giving attention to patient's responsibilities. One should ask who these rights are for, the patient or the advocate."[34]

Not much has changed in Dane County since 1988, when Coroner Clyde Chamberlain was shot to death. In 1991, the City-County Building, in which Chamberlain was shot, was described as "a haven for homeless people after normal business hours. . . . Some of these people are mentally ill. . . . They sleep all over the ground floor and sometimes you can't even get in the doors in the morning." In 1990, the *Capital Times* published a three-part series on Dane County's mentally ill jail inmates, estimated to be between 8 and 15 percent of the jail population. The most common charges leading to their arrests were said to be "lewd and lascivious behavior, defrauding an innkeeper (eating a meal, then not paying for it), disorderly conduct, menacing panhandling, criminal damage to property, loitering or petty theft." A major reason for the jailing of the mentally ill persons, according to the newspaper, was "the strictness of the state's emergency detention law." By 1998, the census of the county jail had again doubled, and the Dane County sheriff observed that "county jails are one of the biggest mental health facilities in the country."[35]

Homicides and other episodes of violence associated with mentally ill persons have continued to occur regularly in Dane County. The most highly publicized episode took place four months after the Chamberlain murder. Laurie Dann, a thirty-year-old woman living in an apartment in Madison, was familiar to both local police and the FBI. She was suspected of stabbing her ex-husband, had harassed and threatened a variety of acquaintances, and was well known in the community for her strange behavior. She was seeing a Madison psychiatrist intermittently. In April, aware that Dann was deteriorating, the psychiatrist considered hospitalizing her but concluded that she did not meet the state's commitment criteria. On May 15, she was questioned by the police when she was found in the apartment building's garbage room, "burrowed into the refuse . . . wrapped in a plastic bag." She was "just looking for things," she said.

Six days later in Winnetka, Illinois, Dann delivered arsenic-laced juice and cookies to the homes of five acquaintances and set fires in a school and a daycare center. Armed with three guns, she then entered a second-grade classroom, where she killed one child and wounded five others. Finally, she seriously wounded a man before killing herself. When the Madison police were asked why they had not detained Dann six days earlier, a spokesman said, "The fact that someone had serious violence in their history and is now acting strangely is not enough. . . . You have to have a pretty strong case."[36]

Another highly publicized Dane County incident occurred in April 1997. Eugene Devoe, diagnosed with schizophrenia, beat a female university student with a large stapler. The newspaper noted that in 1979, he had attacked another female student in the library with an ax, causing severe head injuries. At the time of the second attack, he was apparently not taking medication. Within sixteen months following Devoe's 1997 attack, the following additional tragedies were recorded in Madison:

- Brandon Grady, diagnosed with schizophrenia, used a hammer to kill a woman in a Madison motel.
- Salim Amara, diagnosed with paranoid schizophrenia, dumped a bucket of gasoline onto a random passenger on a Madison bus, then threw a lit match at him. In the resulting fire, six people were injured, "several of them critically."
- Oto Orlik, diagnosed with bipolar disorder, stabbed his daughter to death and tried to kill his wife.
- Renaldo Gettridge, said to be "paranoid and delusional," shot to death an eighteen-year-old man in a parking lot.[37]

That situation existed, and continues to exist, in the county that is widely regarded as having the best public psychiatric services in the United States among all 3,139 counties.

Reform of the Laws

As the effects of the *Lessard* decision grew apparent in the years after its implementation, many people began calling for legal reforms. Among them was Wisconsin's governor, Lee Dreyfus, who "became concerned about the number of obviously mentally ill persons on the streets of the capital who were wandering into the capitol building and into his office."[38] In 1982, the governor appointed an ad hoc committee to explore possible modifications to the commitment statutes; Darold Treffert was a member of the committee. In 1984, a bill was introduced in the state legislature, but support was tepid.

The murders by Bryan Stanley in February 1985 abruptly increased interest in amending the state's mental health laws. Stanley exemplified the problem of a person who was severely mentally ill but who was not being treated, because he did not meet existing criteria for involuntary treatment. One week after the killings, Mary Stanley, Bryan's mother, publicly stated, "If there is any good to come from this, maybe it will be that laws will be changed so that people like [Bryan] can get help in the future. The people are crying for help. Their families are crying for help." A few months later, Gary Stanley, Bryan's brother, testified before the state assembly in favor of the reform legislation. Under the current laws, Gary Stanley said, "his brother essentially was allowed to decide for himself whether he needed help." He added that "his experience with the mental health care system in the state had made him aware of other people like his brother who are 'walking time bombs.'"[39]

It took eleven years for legislation to finally pass and amend the state's mental health laws. Mary Stanley made it her life's work, regularly reminding state legislators and others that her son, like the three men he killed, had been a victim of the *Lessard*-instigated laws. Assemblyman John Medinger, the state representative from La Crosse and a close personal friend of Father Rossiter's, and Senator Peggy Rosen-zweig led the support in the legislature. Roz Libman of the Wisconsin Alliance for the Mentally Ill worked closely with Mary Stanley and other families. But the key to passage was the relentless advocacy of Darold Treffert and the support of the Wisconsin Medical Society.

Opposition to the reforms was substantial. Civil libertarians argued that broadening commitment standards "could lead to people being committed without cause or being held in institutions longer than nec-essary." Some mental health professionals also opposed reform, espe-cially those in Dane County who felt that the proposed legislation implied that their much lauded program was not working. David Goodrick, director of the State Office of Mental Health, argued that the proposed changes "would significantly increase inpatient utiliza-tion, . . . have a dramatically negative fiscal impact on the Department and counties," and be "divisive, polarizing, and damaging to the public mental health system."[40]

The strongest resistance to modifying Wisconsin's mental health laws, however, came from lawyers. Leading the opposition was Thomas Zander, a Milwaukee public defender who did not believe that mental illness was a disease or in fact even existed. A cum laude graduate of the University of Wisconsin and its School of Law, Zander acknowl-edges having been profoundly influenced by Thomas Szasz. As the director of the publicly funded Legal Aid Society of Milwaukee, Zan-der defended over one thousand severely mentally ill individuals to try to prevent their involuntary hospitalization, and he has publicly argued "that non-dangerous people have the right to be mentally ill." He has acknowledged that his own personal lifestyle has influenced his advo-cacy for mentally ill persons. He recalled his distress, as a young gay man coming out of the closet in the late 1960s and 1970s, when some psychiatrists claimed that homosexuality was a mental disease and advocated treatment for it. Zander has been a leader in Milwaukee's gay community and in 1998 became the first person with AIDS to chair the Milwaukee Ryan White Consortium.[41]

In a published interview, Zander maintained that mental illness "is learned behavior that can be unlearned . . . a matter of choice on the part of his clients." After handling "thousands of cases," he could not think of a single example "where involuntary commitment is truly necessary." And involuntary medication, according to Zander, was anathema: "What right does the state have to take over somebody's brain chemistry against their will?" Zander's efforts to block reform of the mental health laws were assisted by other lawyers, especially Dianne Greenley of the Wisconsin Coalition for Advocacy. Greenley, who also expressed doubts about the validity of "the biomedical model" of mental illness, argued that the proposed legislation would "cause personal pain and loss to those subject to unnecessary commitments" and would "create enormous fiscal consequences for the counties."[42]

Despite such opposition, legislation reforming Wisconsin's mental health laws passed in April 1996. The reform established a new standard for involuntary commitment, permitting the hospitalization of individuals with a documented history of mental illness who are in need of treatment and who will likely suffer severe harm if not treated. None of the dire consequences predicted by Zander, Greenley, and other opponents of the legislation came to pass, and in fact the new standard was used only about thirty times each year throughout the state in the first three years following its passage.[43]

Although the new standard was not employed often, Thomas Zander filed a petition in July 2000 to have its constitutionality reviewed by the state courts. The petitioner in the case was Dennis H., a man selected by Zander, who had been diagnosed with schizophrenia for almost thirty years. The man had virtually no awareness of his illness, refused to take medication voluntarily, and had delusional beliefs leading him periodically to refuse to eat or drink anything. During periods when the man had been made to take medication, he had worked part-time, lived in stable housing, and had had a girlfriend. During periods when he had not taken medication, he had been intermittently homeless, violent toward family members, and hospitalized for dehydration and acute kidney failure resulting from his refusal to eat or drink. After the man was forced to accept medication under the new standard, Zander filed a petition that would have allowed the man to again refuse medication. The case was ultimately heard by the Wisconsin Supreme

Court, which in 2002 unanimously upheld the new standard as constitutional. In issuing the ruling, one justice noted, "For family members and friends, a loved one's refusal of timely treatment can result in an agonizing and helpless vigil as that individual's mental, emotional and physical condition deteriorates."[44]

Whatever Happened to Ms. Lessard?

Today in Wisconsin, mental health services for persons with severe psychiatric disorders vary widely from county to county. Homeless persons talking to themselves are prevalent in every city and in many medium-sized towns. County jails and state prisons continue to be overcrowded, in part because they house so many prisoners with severe mental illnesses. The media regularly report on homicides and other tragedies involving mentally ill persons who are not receiving treatment.

Deinstitutionalization eliminated most long-term psychiatric beds in the state. The city of Milwaukee had approximately four thousand such beds at the time of the *Lessard* decision; today it has about one hundred. Many of the patients who would have occupied those beds are now among the homeless and the incarcerated. Others, estimated to number about five hundred, are in nursing homes. One for-profit nursing home, described by the *Milwaukee Journal Sentinel*, was virtually a small psychiatric hospital with 101 residents diagnosed with schizophrenia and other severe mental disorders. A former manager said that "the only stimulation a lot of those people got was when one resident would scream at another."[45]

Where are all of the other patients who once would have been in the hospitals? A March 2006 series in the *Milwaukee Journal Sentinel* provided harsh answers. It described hundreds of mentally ill individuals "living in illegal group homes and rooming houses—many of them filthy and dangerous, some deadly—which have sprung up as stealth mental hospitals to replace county wards." Some of the homes had "no running water, no heat, rats, roaches, broken smoke detectors and faulty wiring." In one house, "a 52-year-old woman with schizophrenia . . .

was dead for more than three days . . . before the landlady smelled a horrible odor coming from her room." In another, the reporters found a fifty-nine-year-old woman with diabetes and schizophrenia "lying on a bare mattress soaked in her urine," surrounded by "mounds of spent toilet paper."[46]

The newspaper series also reported on the victimization of the mentally ill. One man with schizophrenia, "well-known for walking the neighborhood with Bible in hand, quoting from Scripture," was beaten to death. Landlords were said to sometimes abuse residents. "Building inspectors have found people begging on the streets for food because they don't get enough from landlords who take their disability checks, leaving them with next to nothing." Asked for his thoughts on the situation, Zander, now retired, said, "People with mental illnesses have been left out in the cold. Literally. It's inhumane. I never said, 'Let's close all mental hospitals.' I said, 'Let's close all the ones with locks on the door.'"[47]

Onalaska has never completely recovered from the Bryan Stanley murders. Articles about the victims' families are carried by the newspaper on major anniversaries of the tragedy. Rose Hammes misses her father and regrets that he was not alive for her college graduation. She believes that Bryan Stanley "got off" and has vigorously opposed his requests for release from the hospital.[48]

In December 2005, on a cold, snowy day, I visited Mary Stanley. She is a petite, eighty-three-year-old, very pleasant woman who has lived alone since her husband died. When I arrived, she was shoveling the walk so that I wouldn't fall. She has six children besides Bryan and sixteen grandchildren. She is proud of her role in getting Wisconsin's mental health laws reformed in order that other families do not have to suffer. She noted, "Our family was a victim of the laws too."

Bryan Stanley is still a patient at Mendota Mental Health Institute. He has been there for twenty-two years, at a cost of almost $700 per day; thus, his hospital costs alone total 5.5 million Wisconsin tax dollars. In addition, he receives a VA disability check of $1,900 per month, which totals an additional half million dollars. His schizophrenia has been in remission for many years on an antipsychotic medication, clozapine, and he holds a part-time job in the community. In 2006, using some of his VA disability funds, he published a book promoting the creation of a national park in a scenic area in western Wisconsin, and he continues to be intensely interested in environmental causes. His requests for release from the hospital have been rejected five times, yet he remains hopeful. He did not agree to an interview, understandably not interested in doing anything that might publicize his case.

There are indications that Bryan Stanley does not fully understand and accept the fact that he has schizophrenia. Shortly after his trial in 1985, he wrote that his problems had developed because he "was given some bad advice by two priests at a time when it did the most damage." He believed that he had been "brainwashed." Four years later, he wrote to a newspaper, "It's hard to accept that I am mentally ill, and it will take another episode to prove to me that I am mentally ill."[49]

Stanley is aware that he will never be released from the hospital unless he is taking medication, and so he has taken it willingly most of the time. Eight years after the murders, however, he "began wondering if he would develop symptoms if he went off medication." Despite entreaties from hospital staff, he refused to take it for several days. When asked to list his two goals for achieving discharge, he gave as number one to "go off my medication."[50] Today, there is probably nobody who knows Bryan Stanley well who expects that he would continue taking medication voluntarily if he were released from the hospital.

Alberta Lessard, the face behind the name that changed Wisconsin's mental health laws, agreed to see me. We met in early March 2006, on a clear, crisp day when winds from Lake Michigan were blowing through Milwaukee's residential streets, reminding residents why so many of their neighbors had not yet returned from the south. She greeted me pleasantly, white-haired but looking younger than her eighty-five years, despite her use of a walker, a consequence of a recent fall.[51]

Her small, ground-floor apartment was clean, orderly, and dominated by a writing table. She was somewhat shy until I asked about politics, at which point she effloresced and talked excitedly about her projects. Her piles of news clippings rested next to a box with perhaps twenty envelopes addressed to various federal, state, and local officials and to the editors of various newspapers. She acknowledged being one of the best customers of the U.S. Postal Service and complained that stamps usurp a disproportionate share of her monthly SSDI check. A television set on the table is usually tuned to news programs, she says, especially C-SPAN.

She proudly displayed her letters, which were well written and covered a variety of local, state, and national issues. She recognized the difficulty in getting politicians' attention, so she often addressed them by nicknames or put information on the envelopes to pique the recipients' interest. She showed me a letter addressed to State Attorney General Peggy Lautenschlager, whom she addressed as "Dilly Dallying Sluggish Slacker." Another letter was addressed to James Sensenbrenner, who represents Ms. Lessard's district in Congress and is apparently a frequent recipient of her missives; as chairman of the House Committee on the Judiciary, Sensenbrenner advertises himself as a "watchdog," but Ms. Lessard addressed him as "mad dog." President George Bush, she said, is evil incarnate and "should be tried as a war criminal."

The purpose of the letters, said Ms. Lessard, is to expose corruption, which she believes is ubiquitous. She proudly claims that her letters have exposed "more than a dozen politicians" who were forced out of office as a result of her efforts, although she readily gives credit to others for helping. She is knowledgeable about local, state, and federal laws and in previous years filed many suits against various officials. In the dismissal of one suit, the court noted,

She seeks judgments declaring unconstitutional several statutes ranging from Wisconsin's disorderly conduct statute to the state's welfare system. . . . She seeks to declare "all elections from the time of Richard Nixon's illegal." . . . It is clear from her complaint that the plaintiff wishes to challenge nearly every facet of government in existence today.[52]

I asked Ms. Lessard about her life prior to the suit filed on her behalf in 1971. She talked readily about growing up during the Great Depression, when "we made our own soap and clothes." Despite the family's poverty, she remembered her childhood fondly as a tomboy with five siblings. As a teacher, she received outstanding ratings, she said, and even helped teach student teachers in the Marquette University Reading Center. When asked why she had lost her job, she said that the school board had given no reason other than that she had "challenged the system." She also explained that "the union tried to break into [her] apartment." She clearly remembered being involuntarily hospitalized; once there, she called lawyers at Milwaukee Legal Services, who filed a class action suit, and the rest is legal history.

Ms. Lessard's life since 1972 has not been easy. She has never been able to return to work and has had to live frugally on the monthly SSDI check that she receives, she says, "because they say I am mentally ill." In the months following the *Lessard* decision, she appeared regularly as a spectator in the courtroom of Judge Myron Gordon, one member of the three-judge panel who ruled in her favor. According to Judge Gordon, Ms. Lessard "would stand up in court in the middle of the hearings and give her opinion." On several occasions, she had to be escorted by bailiffs from the courtroom; on one occasion, she was even driven by bailiffs to the County Mental Health Center for a psychiatric evaluation.[53]

Ms. Lessard acknowledges that over the years she gave local officials "a few problems." She says she landed in jail "dozens of times," but always "on trumped-up charges." The Milwaukee County court records that are still available reveal ten charges against Ms. Lessard between 1977 and 2003; they include theft (trying to steal a court file); battery (striking a court clerk who said that a requested record would not be available until the following day because of a computer breakdown); and criminal damage to property (breaking the glass door of the district attorney's office and entering it after the office had closed for the day). She was also convicted of abusing the 911 emergency call line and setting off the apartment smoke alarm "to see if the Fire Department vehicles would come with red lights and siren, and to see if they would break down her door and rescue her." On one occasion when the police came to her apartment to investigate, she threw tomatoes at them from her second-story window.

Some of the charges against Ms. Lessard have been more serious. In 1999, at age seventy-nine, she was charged with making "repeated threats to shoot school board members with a gun, and to go into schools and shoot students and faculty members. . . . The defendant claimed to have a gun in her purse and reached inside as if she was retrieving something." On another occasion, she drove past a police car stopped at a red light; with the officer in pursuit with lights flashing and siren blaring, she led him on a four-mile chase through downtown Milwaukee as she ran six more red lights. When she was finally stopped, she said, "I did pretty good, I went through all those red lights and did not have an accident, I'm a good driver." She was also charged with driving without a license.[54]

Ms. Lessard's behavior has gotten her evicted from apartments "five or six times." As a consequence, she spent periods living on the streets. She spent two months homeless in Milwaukee one winter, which is not, she readily acknowledged, a good time to be homeless there.

The most difficult part of Ms. Lessard's life, however, has been constant harassment and persecution. For more than forty years, she says, she has been subjected to electronic surveillance and break-ins of her apartment. The people follow her, spy on her, steal her mail, and mess up things in her apartment. She says they break into her place "nine out of ten times" when she goes out and even enter at night when she is asleep. Recently, they even took the covers off her bed and put them on the floor while she slept. Such harassment has been unending, month after month and year after year. When I asked who the people are and why they do it, she said it is, of course, public officials who are angry at her for exposing their corruption.

When I asked Ms. Lessard about psychiatric treatment, she acknowledged that since 1972 she had been briefly involuntarily hospitalized several times. She had never agreed to take psychiatric medication, she said, and only took it "when forced"; "it made me sick and dizzy and I could hardly walk." She is convinced that taking psychiatric medications is the primary cause of schizophrenia and has nothing but disdain for psychiatry, calling it "the most lucrative of all forms of witchcraft."

In both humanitarian and economic terms, what might have happened to Alberta Lessard had her lawyers in 1971 insisted that she receive treatment rather than filing suit to effectively block treatment? The chances are reasonably good that she would have responded to medication if she had been adequately treated. She might have returned to teaching, contributed to society, paid taxes, and led a much different life.

But Ms. Lessard would never have accepted treatment voluntarily. She adamantly believed then, and continues to believe today, that she has never been mentally ill and thus there was no need for her to take psychiatric medication. When I asked her directly whether she ever considered that she might have schizophrenia, she responded, "Absolutely not. I never had any of the symptoms." When a newspaper reporter recently asked her what effect her famous lawsuit has had on psychiatric services in Wisconsin, she responded, "In some ways my case made things worse. There are lots of people out on the street who have to get arrested just to get some help. That's not any too nice."[55]

7 | God Does Not
Take Medication

Lack of insight is so frequently present in schizophrenia (and some other psychoses as well) that it is unreasonable to expect patients to always recognize or accept their need for treatment on a voluntary basis. If we can agree with the premise that the liberty to be psychotic is no freedom at all, then we can begin to examine some of the current plights of the mentally ill patients.

STEPHEN RACHLIN, 1974

Malcoum Tate heard God almost every day. God had given him a mission—to rid the world of evil people—and Malcoum was determined to carry out that mission. Malcoum focused on the evil in his own family, especially his niece, N'Zinga, and his mother. He repeatedly told his mother, "Mama, you just remember now that when I'm killing you, it's not really me who is doing it but God."

Herb Mullin received "cosmic emanations" that gave him instructions. Later, he realized that it was God speaking to him and that he had been anointed a prophet. Herb believed that he had been appointed by God to sacrifice others to prevent a major earthquake, and he carried out his mission to the best of his ability.

Bryan Stanley also had a mission from God. He was Elijah, sent "to purify the Church" and "to save the world from war, communism and sin." He received explicit instructions from the Virgin Mary. In killing

111

"three devils," he said, he was acting as "a soldier of Christ" and expected to be rewarded for his actions.

Anosognosia

Malcoum Tate, Herb Mullin, and Bryan Stanley shared three important attributes. Each believed he was on a God-appointed mission; each had schizophrenia; and each had no awareness of, or insight into, his illness. It is this last attribute that makes schizophrenia the most misunderstood, most difficult to treat, and most pernicious of all human psychiatric disorders.

The fact that some people with severe psychiatric disorders lack insight into their illness has been noted throughout history. In a seventeenth-century play by Thomas Dekker, a character says, "That proves you mad because you know it not." A nineteenth-century article noted, "Generally, insane people do not regard themselves as insane, and consequently can see no reason for their confinement." Emil Kraepelin, commenting in the early twentieth century on insane people's lack of awareness of illness, quoted a patient: "Whoever thinks that I am mad, is himself mad." More recently, H. G. Woodley, the pseudonym of Herbert George Wilkins, who had been psychiatrically hospitalized, wrote, "Indeed, the one and only thing that is typical of *all* lunatics is their inability to comprehend that they are insane. . . . To tell them that they are insane is really wasting words, for they at once pity you in your great ignorance in thinking such a thing possible."[1]

Woodley's assertion that "*all* lunatics" lack awareness of their illness is not correct. Multiple studies, using a variety of measures, have suggested that approximately half of all individuals with schizophrenia and bipolar disorder are aware of their illness. Most of them take their medication as needed. The other half, however, have impaired awareness of their illness. One study, for example, reported that 57 percent of individuals with schizophrenia "had moderate to severe unawareness of having a mental disorder." Patients with bipolar disorder, especially those in a manic phase and/or with delusions and hallucinations, show similar levels of impairment, but there is an important difference. Individuals with bipolar disorder are more likely to regain insight once they are treated or otherwise go into spontaneous remission, whereas those with schizophrenia are less likely to do so.[2] Treating individuals like Malcoum Tate, Herb Mullin, and Bryan Stanley with medication will sometimes improve their insight, but more often it will not.

"The Loss of Insight"

Laura Van Tosh, forty-three, of Silver Spring, Maryland, works as a community liaison with inpatients at Springfield Hospital Center and is a mental health policy consultant who has spent many years as a vocal consumer advocate at the national level. "I lost insight about eight years ago when I had a relapse," Laura says, "I had actually thought I had 'recovered' from my mental illness when, in fact, I had been slowly descending into madness. I found myself in the middle of the street, barefoot, and at risk.

"The lack of insight on my part, coupled with my psychiatrist's inexperience, made insight the pivotal issue in the crisis. Unfortunately, no one knew enough to stop the wheels from turning. I learned later that communication with loved ones and others with mental illness is an absolute necessity in maintaining my recovery. My family and friends know about my illness and they support me as much as possible in advance of a crisis.

"The loss of insight resulted in my being involuntarily committed and while I had been a staunch opponent of such forceful measures, involuntary commitment actually saved my life."

I. S. Levine, "Insight: The key piece in recovery's puzzle," **Schizophrenia Digest,** *fall 2004, pp. 33–34.*

When confronted by people who exhibit no awareness of their illness, we typically assume that they are in denial. Denial is a psychological mechanism whereby an individual, consciously or unconsciously, *chooses* to not acknowledge something. Denial, according to Sigmund

Freud, is used by everyone and has been invoked to explain all manner of forgetting. People with schizophrenia and bipolar disorder are as capable of using denial as anyone else, and given the unpleasantness of these diseases, they have great incentive for doing so.

However, when people like Malcoum Tate, Herb Mullin, and Bryan Stanley deny that anything is wrong with them, we now understand that this usually reflects more than denial. Rather, it reflects an anatomical impairment of the brain circuits we use to think about ourselves. It is a variant of what neurologists refer to as "anosognosia," a term coined in 1914 and meaning "lack of knowledge of disease."

"Anosognosia" was first used to describe individuals who had become paralyzed following a stroke but who denied that they were paralyzed. Examples of this phenomenon include the following:

- A man who had suffered a stroke was asked what was wrong with his paralyzed arm. "It's just a little stiff—from cold or something," he replied. When asked why he couldn't raise it, he replied, "I have a shirt on."
- A woman with paralysis of her left arm was asked to raise her arm. Instead, she raised her left leg. When this was pointed out to her, she said, "Oh, some people call it an arm, some a leg. What's the difference!"
- The best-known individual who had anosognosia following a stroke was former Supreme Court Justice William Douglas, who became paralyzed on his left side. According to one account, "he initially dismissed the paralysis as a myth, and weeks later he was still inviting reporters to go on hiking expeditions with him."[3]

Individuals who suffer strokes and deny the resultant paralysis illustrate important characteristics of anosognosia. Affected individuals sometimes deny their deficits and make up stories—called confabulations—to explain their disability. They also exhibit a lack of concern and a lack of emotional response. In *Descartes' Error*, the neurologist Antonio Damasio described it as follows:

No less dramatic than the oblivion that anosognosic patients have regarding their sick limbs is the lack of concern they show for their overall situation, the lack of emotion they exhibit, the lack of feeling they report when questioned about it. . . . The lack of direct update on the real state of body and person is nothing less than astounding.

Such observations led Damasio to call anosognosia "one of the most eccentric neuropsychological presentations one is likely to encounter." Similarly, in *The Man Who Mistook His Wife for a Hat*, Oliver Sacks said of anosognosia, "It is singularly difficult, for even the most sensitive observer, to picture the inner state . . . for this is almost unimaginably remote from anything he himself has ever known."[4]

In cases of anosognosia caused by strokes, people's awareness of their deficit often improves as their brain function improves. In other cases, as when the condition is caused by Alzheimer's disease, anosognosia is permanent. In the earliest stages of Alzheimer's disease, those affected are aware that their memory is failing. Studies of anosognosia in Alzheimer's patients have shown that it is more severe in those who have had the disease longer and also in individuals who have more cognitive and behavioral impairments.[5] And, like the stroke victims described above, most individuals with Alzheimer's disease are remarkably unconcerned about the deficits or their consequences.

Like Alzheimer's patients, some individuals with schizophrenia possess an awareness of their illness in the earliest stages, only to lose that awareness as the disease progresses. One newspaper report describes a young woman in Oregon who walked in a circle all day, "convinced that was the only way to stop aliens from entering her body." She then called home and told her mother that she thought she was becoming "insane." As her symptoms intensified, she later explained, "I lost my awareness of the illness." In another case, a sixteen-year-old young man realized that he was becoming psychotic. Without saying anything to his family, he went to the local medical library and diagnosed himself with schizophrenia before anyone else knew. He later also lost all awareness of his illness.[6]

The Localization of Anosognosia

Researchers using neuroimaging and neuropsychological techniques have increased our understanding of the physical location in the brain of anosognosia. The studies report that anosognosia is much more likely to occur following damage to the right, nondominant half of the brain. In one study, it occurred four times more frequently following strokes to the right hemisphere than after strokes to the left hemisphere. In Alzheimer's disease, patients with more severe anosognosia also show more evidence of damage to the right side of the brain. Studies of patients with strokes and other brain injuries suggest that damage to areas in the frontal and parietal lobes is most likely to lead to anosognosia.[7]

The frontal and parietal lobes and the connections between them are the areas that also appear to be primarily affected in individuals with schizophrenia who have anosognosia. At least five studies have reported that patients who lack awareness of their illness have more abnormalities in specific frontal lobe areas when compared with those who are aware. Other studies have found correlations between lack of awareness and the parietal lobe, and one study reported that individuals with schizophrenia who lack awareness of their illness have smaller brains in general.[8] The anatomical basis of anosognosia, however, should not be oversimplified. Most brain functions utilize circuits involving multiple brain areas, and this is certainly true for anosognosia. Thus, there is no single "anosognosia center"; rather, self-awareness is a product of a complex circuit prominently involving areas in the frontal and parietal lobes, the connections between them, and other brain areas.

The Consequences of Anosognosia

Malcoum Tate did not take medication, because God did not need it. "Hell, no," he would say, "I won't take it, I don't need no medicine." At times, he expressed a belief that the medication was poison.

Herb Mullin refused to take medication because prophets of God did not need it. Even today he continues to refuse, convinced that nothing is wrong with him. He even wonders whether it was the Thorazine he took during his initial hospitalization that *caused* his homicidal behavior.

Bryan Stanley refused to take medication, despite excellent responses to it during his initial hospitalizations. As Isaiah, he too did not need it. If Bryan Stanley were to be released from the hospital today and given the option of whether or not to continue taking medication, chances are that he would not do so.

The choices Tate, Mullin, and Stanley made were eminently logical, considering their condition. Their behavior strongly suggests that all three men had severe anosognosia, damage to the parts of the brain that govern self-awareness. The same disease process that produced their symptoms of schizophrenia likely caused this damage. Each man was unaware that he was sick and convinced that nothing was wrong with him. Given their beliefs, why should they have taken medicine?

A refusal to take medication is a common outcome for individuals with schizophrenia and bipolar disorder who have anosognosia. Over one hundred studies of medication refusal have been conducted on individuals with schizophrenia, and the rate of refusal ranges between 40 and 50 percent. Medication refusal occurs commonly among the 400,000 individuals with severe psychiatric disorders who are most problematic and is almost universal among the 40,000 who are overtly dangerous. Joseph McEvoy, one of the foremost psychiatric researchers on this issue, summarized compliance studies as follows:

Approximately 50% of patients will take their medications as prescribed with little or no support required. An additional 35% of patients will comply if provided with supervision and support. The remaining 15% of patients will do anything they can to avoid taking medications under any circumstances, and may require coercion to remain compliant.

In one study, 12 percent "adamantly refused to take medication at all, and equated the drugs with poison." In another study, 14 percent refused because of paranoid thinking and "deep-seated delusional beliefs about their medications." The nonadherence rates among individuals with bipolar disorder are reported to be almost as high as for schizophrenia.[9]

The reasons why individuals with severe psychiatric disorders do not take medication as prescribed can include dislike of drug side effects, the high cost of medication, problems with substance abuse, and a poor relationship with the treating psychiatrist. But in virtually every study done on this problem, anosognosia remains the most prominently reported reason. For example, in one study linking lack of awareness to nonadherence, "the participants [with schizophrenia] who were more aware of their mental illnesses and of the beneficial effects of medication were more likely to be compliant with their prescribed medication." In a large national study, it was reported that "patients who lacked awareness had significantly longer episodes of antipsychotic nonadherence [and] were more likely to completely cease taking the antipsychotic medication."[10]

It should be emphasized that many individuals take medication despite their anosognosia. They may do so to please their family or their treating professionals or simply because they generally do whatever doctors ask them to do. Other patients will take medication because they have learned that whenever they do not, they end up in the hospital. They may have little awareness of their illness, but they recognize the causal link.

Lack of awareness of illness is the most common cause of relapse and rehospitalization. In one study, "only 8 percent of patients with insight required hospitalization for their relapse, in contrast to 50 percent of those without insight." Another large study found a "direct relationship between measures of partial compliance and risk of hospitalization: the lower the level of compliance, the greater the risk of hospitalization."[11]

Refusal to take medication also markedly increases chances that individuals with schizophrenia or bipolar disorder will become homeless or be incarcerated. A study of individuals discharged from a Massachusetts state psychiatric hospital reported that 63 percent of those who became homeless did not take medication. Other studies have also found medication refusal to be a leading risk factor for homelessness among individuals with schizophrenia. In addition, medication refusal and substance abuse were reported to be "two highly significant predictors of arrest" among mentally ill individuals. In one study, twenty-one out of sixty-five patients released from an Ohio state psychiatric hospital were arrested within six months of release; "psychotropic medication had been prescribed upon their discharge from the state hospital, but the residents failed to take their medication."[12]

"The Client Has to Make That Request"

In 2003, Jermaine Berry, age twenty, shot two Boston-area police officers. Berry had been diagnosed with schizophrenia and hospitalized six times in the preceding five years. He had set fire to his family home, threatened to jump off the roof, and told his parents, "I am God. Nothing can kill me." He responded well to medication while hospitalized but frequently refused to take it when not hospitalized, consistently demonstrating little awareness of his illness. Despite this, the mental health system treated him as if he were fully competent to make rational decisions. When members of his family pleaded with hospital officials to keep him longer, they were told, "There's nothing we can do; he's at the age where he can sign himself out." And when asked why mental health officials had terminated Berry's case manager, who was providing some support while he was an outpatient, a spokesperson said, "We could have maintained contact with him, *but the client has to make that request*" (emphasis added).

From E. Barry and F. Stockman, **Boston Globe,**
January 3, 2003.

The most serious consequence of anosognosia, and the medication refusal that so frequently accompanies it, is violent behavior. In one study of psychiatric outpatients, "71 percent of the violent patients . . . had problems with medication compliance, compared with only 17 percent of those without hostile behaviors." Another large study of almost two thousand individuals with schizophrenia demonstrated that those who were nonadherent with medications were twice as likely to commit violent acts and also twice as likely to be arrested, rehospitalized, or victimized by criminal acts.[13]

At least five studies have linked increased anosognosia to increased violent behavior. Presumably this stems from the fact that anosognosia causes medication refusal, which in turn leads to violent behavior. In an Ohio study of 226 patients with schizophrenia, half of whom had been violent and half of whom had not, those who had been violent demonstrated significantly less insight on testing and also had an "inability to appreciate the relationship of illness to crime." A study in New York assessed insight in sixty men with severe psychiatric disorders, half of whom had a history of violent behavior and half of whom did not. In the violent group, insight was significantly impaired compared with the nonviolent group. Similar findings linking lack of awareness directly to violent behavior have been reported in studies in Israel, Sweden, England, Ireland, and Spain; in the last, "the single variable that best predicted violence was [impaired] insight into psychotic symptoms."[14]

Unaware of Unawareness

Given what is known about impaired brain function in individuals with schizophrenia and bipolar disorder, including the fact that it may produce anosognosia, it is understandable why Malcoum Tate, Herb Mullin, and Bryan Stanley refused medication. Since research on anosognosia in psychiatric patients is only two decades old, it is also understandable that most laws governing mentally ill persons have not yet incorporated the results of this research. Among mental health authorities and state legislators, there is widespread unawareness of unawareness.

The architects of the Lanterman-Petris-Short Act and the *Lessard* decision clearly demonstrated this deficit. In California, Assemblyman Frank Lanterman explicitly rejected any concept of anosognosia:

For too many years the presumption has been that a mentally disturbed individual will not admit to being "sick" and will not accept recommended treatment. Therefore, it is thought necessary to contain him so he cannot escape from treatment. This is sometimes justified on the grounds that "the individual will later recognize it was all for his own good." To me this concept is indefensible.[15]

Lanterman's assumption was that all psychiatric patients are competent to choose whether or not they wish to take medication or to be otherwise treated. In testimony before the California Senate Select Committee, Kenneth Springer, the foreman of the jury that convicted Herb Mullin, had the final say on Lanterman's assumption: "I think that this [LPS] Act presumes that a mental patient will voluntarily commit himself for mental treatment. Senator, I think that [only] sane persons volunteer for medical treatment."[16]

Those involved in the *Lessard* decision also seemed unaware of anosognosia and assumed that psychiatrically ill individuals possessed both the competency and the right to make treatment decisions. The three judges who wrote the decision stated, "Persons in need of hospitalization for mental illness should be allowed the choice of whether to undergo hospitalization and treatment or not, unless the state can prove that the person is unable to make decisions about hospitalization because of the nature of the illness." When courts in Milwaukee began using insight as a measure of being "unable to make decisions," the public defender Thomas Zander protested bitterly. The *Lessard* decision, Zander said, "proclaims that non-dangerous people have the right to be mentally ill."[17]

The three judges who rendered the *Lessard* decision also compared psychiatric illnesses to physical illnesses. "Persons in need of hospitalization for physical ailments are allowed the choice of whether to undergo hospitalization and treatment or not," they wrote, and then added, "The same should be true of persons in need of treatment for mental illness." People with a diseased heart or kidney can, of course, make rational decisions regarding their treatment. What the judges seemed unaware of is that some people with a diseased brain are no longer capable of making rational decisions, because their disease affects the part of the body used for such decisions.[18]

Here, then, are the roots of deinstitutionalization's failure. Most laws governing the treatment of mentally ill individuals assume that such individuals are competent to accept or reject treatment, with the sole exception of obvious dementia. Yet, contemporary research has established that up to half of all individuals with severe psychiatric disorders are not competent to assess their own need for treatment. The consequences of this misunderstanding have led to increasing numbers of mentally ill individuals who are homeless, incarcerated, and victimized, and increasing numbers of individuals who commit homicides and other violent acts. This misunderstanding underlies one of the great social disasters of late twentieth-century America.

8 | The Consequences of Unconstrained Civil Liberties: Homeless, Incarcerated, and Victimized

Uninformed calls to protect civil liberties betray a profound misunderstanding of that term. There is nothing "civil" about leaving people lost to disease to live homeless on the streets, suffering rape and victimization. There is nothing "right" about leaving someone untreated and psychotic, rendering them incapable of discerning whether they are attacking a CIA operative or their own mother.

MARY ZDANOWICZ, 2006

The Lanterman-Petris-Short Act and the *Lessard* decision profoundly affected mental health laws in other states. Washington State copied LPS in 1974, and the following year Massachusetts, New York, and Pennsylvania introduced legislation "closely patterned after the success of LPS." By 1988, it was said that "most state commitment statutes today are modeled after California's Lanterman-Petris-Short Act." Before the *Lessard* decision, only nine states used "dangerousness" as the sole criterion for involuntary psychiatric hospitalization. By 1980, "every state had changed its statute to restrict hospitalization to persons who were dangerous to themselves or others . . . or had interpreted its preexisting statute in a way so as to save it from being found unconstitutional."[1]

LPS and *Lessard* were bellwethers for what was to come. Throughout the 1970s and early 1980s, civil rights lawyers challenged mental

123

health statutes in almost every state. Although their legal strategies differed, their common goal was to make involuntary commitment and involuntary treatment as difficult as possible and ultimately to close the state psychiatric hospitals. This flood of litigation had inevitable consequences throughout the United States for the severely mentally ill individuals who were then released from state mental hospitals and for all those individuals who became severely mentally ill in the decades that followed. Among the most important consequences were homelessness, incarceration, and victimization. These consequences are clearly visible today, especially among the subset of mentally ill persons who are unaware of their illness and who do not take medication. These persons are the flotsam of the earlier legal deluge.

Homelessness

Although there have always been people called hobos or tramps in the United States, the rise of mass homelessness closely parallels the emptying of the nation's public psychiatric hospitals. Beginning in the early 1970s, increasing numbers of homeless individuals, many of whom were overtly psychotic, were visible on urban streets. In the 1980s, they were politicized, provoking major debates regarding their numbers, their origin, and the relative responsibility of local, state, and federal governments for their care. By the turn of this century, the homeless were no longer causes célèbres, having quietly blended into urban landscapes like abandoned cars and rundown buildings.

A 2005 federal survey reported that approximately 500,000 single people and 250,000 families are homeless at any given time. Multiple studies have reported that at least one-third of homeless men and two-thirds of homeless women have serious psychiatric disorders, often exacerbated by alcohol and/or drug abuse. These numbers suggest that there are at present approximately 175,000 homeless men and women who are seriously mentally ill. Among the hardcore homeless, the "permanent street dwellers," the incidence of severe mental illness is much higher; a 2003 study in Miami, for example, found that "every one of them was mentally ill." The lives of these people are bleak; studies have shown that many of the hardcore homeless use garbage cans as their primary food source.[2]

Mentally Ill Homeless Persons Who Achieve Fame

Most mentally ill homeless persons live and die in obscurity. Occasionally, one achieves transient fame, sometimes in life but more often in death. For example, in 1982, Rebecca Smith froze to death in a cardboard box on the streets of New York; the media featured her life when it became known that she had been valedictorian of her college class before becoming psychiatrically ill. In 1993, Yetta Adams, diagnosed with schizophrenia, froze to death on a bench directly across the street from the headquarters of the Department of Housing and Urban Development (HUD) in Washington; Henry Cisneros, HUD secretary, joined the crowd to see what had happened and later wrote, "Yetta Adams' death jarred me and all my colleagues at HUD."*

Perhaps the most famous mentally ill homeless person was Larry Hogue, diagnosed with bipolar disorder and cocaine addiction and known as the "madman of 96th Street." For almost a decade, he terrorized a neighborhood on New York's Upper West Side, setting fires under cars, throwing stones through car windows, masturbating in front of children, pushing a schoolgirl into the path of an oncoming truck, and threatening to roast and eat a woman's dog. He was regularly featured by the New York media because, despite at least nine arrests and thirty brief psychiatric hospitalizations, officials claimed that the state's commitment laws did not allow Hogue to be involuntarily hospitalized or treated long-term. Yet during these years, he continued to receive $3,000 each month in disability benefits from the Veterans Administration.

*H. G. Cisneros, "The lonely death on my doorstep,"
Washington Post, December 5, 1993.

Officials nationwide routinely deny the local origins of their homeless problem and claim that the homeless people in their city came from somewhere else. Such claims have been made not only for warm-weather cities like Miami and Los Angeles but also for cold-weather cities. In Madison, Wisconsin, an official asserted that homeless persons had migrated there because "they have heard that Madison is a nice place to live." Incredibly, even officials in Fargo, North Dakota, have claimed that their city has become a magnet for the homeless. Studies suggest otherwise; for example, in Los Angeles a survey found that 78 percent of homeless persons had lived there prior to becoming homeless.[3]

The true origin of homeless mentally ill persons is no mystery. In Massachusetts, 27 percent of patients discharged from a public psychiatric hospital became homeless within six months of discharge. In a similar study in Ohio, the figure was 36 percent. In New York, 38 percent of psychiatric patients had "no known address" six months after their release.[4] Having been treated with medications while hospitalized, most of these individuals were psychiatrically stable when they left the hospital but then failed to seek follow-up care, because they did not believe they were sick. Studies of mentally ill persons in Massachusetts and New York have shown, not surprisingly, a strong correlation between not taking medication and becoming homeless.[5]

That correlation has been shown to be true even in some highly regarded community treatment programs that are designed to minimize it. In one such program in Philadelphia, 11 percent of the patients became homeless.[6] Severely mentally ill individuals in these programs are *encouraged* to take medications but usually not *made* to do so. In most states, the laws are such that patients cannot be made to take medication unless and until they are proven to be dangerous. Thus, even in the best treatment programs, mentally ill individuals are allowed to deteriorate, their right to do so protected by state laws.

A memorable example of deterioration of a severely mentally ill homeless person was reported in 2005 in Augusta, Maine. Randy Reed, a forty-three-year-old man, dug out a cave-like home for himself on the steep bank of the Kennebec River. Mental health outreach workers and police were aware of Reed and offered him help, but he refused; Maine's strict commitment laws do not allow for involuntary assistance except under extreme circumstances. Reed continued enlarging his home to the point that it eventually undermined a city parking lot, causing it to sag. Reed was then deemed eligible for psychiatric commitment because of the danger posed to the parking lot, not to Reed himself.[7]

Similar scenarios are now common across the country. As a Miami police officer noted, "Seeing another human being living like an animal in America, it just shouldn't be like that. It gets frustrating not being able to do anything legally to help." Another person who works with the homeless described it as follows: "Some of us look on this as an ethical problem. A society that will not care for those least able to care for themselves is an immoral society."[8]

In addition to being inhumane, leaving mentally ill individuals untreated and homeless in the community has consequences for other members of society. A California study found that homeless individuals who had a history of a previous psychiatric hospitalization had almost three times more felony convictions than homeless persons with no psychiatric history. Similarly, a New York study reported that, among mentally ill persons who were homeless and thus unlikely to be taking medications, "the rate of violent crimes was 40 times higher and the rate of nonviolent crimes was 27 times higher" than among mentally ill persons who were in stable housing and thus more likely to be taking medication to control their symptoms.[9]

An especially sobering example of a crime committed disproportionately by homeless mentally ill persons is pushing strangers onto the tracks of a subway. A study in New York City reported that 41 percent of such perpetrators were homeless and 59 percent were psychotic at the time they committed the crime.

- **April 1999:** In New York, Julio Perez, homeless and not being treated for his schizophrenia, pushed Edgar Rivera onto the tracks in front of an oncoming subway train. Perez had a history of violent behavior, including attempted murder, and "had spent the day of the attack roaming city streets, convinced people were trying to kill him." Rivera lost both legs but survived the attack. In a remarkable statement while hospitalized, Rivera said, "I have no legs, but at least I have my mind. This guy doesn't have that. I think I'm ahead."[10]

Events like this are a consequence of unconstrained civil liberties: when we protect the rights of severely mentally ill people so stringently that they cannot be treated, we infringe on the rights of other members of society, sometimes with tragic outcomes.

Incarceration

A massive increase in the number of mentally ill persons in jails and prisons is another consequence of emptying public psychiatric hospitals and then passing laws that prevent the treatment of individuals after their release. As was noted in chapter 6, Lionel Penrose demonstrated in 1939 that psychiatric hospital and prison populations were inversely correlated—as one decreased, the other increased—and other researchers have subsequently replicated this relationship. It has also been widely observed by jail officials at the local level; for example, when the Georgia Mental Health Institute in suburban Atlanta closed in the late 1990s, the local "jail's population of inmates with mental illness increased dramatically."[11]

Throughout the United States, the increase in mentally ill persons in jails and prisons grew apparent as deinstitutionalization became more widespread. A 1975 study in Denver found that "the number of psychotic persons encountered in the jail was striking" and noted a widespread belief among jail personnel "that there had been a marked increase in the number of severely mentally disturbed individuals entering the jail in recent years."[12]

At present, opinions differ regarding the percentage of severely mentally ill individuals who are inmates in the nation's jails and prisons. Conservative estimates put the figure at between 7 and 10 percent.

A widely quoted, but methodologically questionable, federal study reported that 16 percent of individuals in local jails and state prisons self-reported having a "mental condition" or having been psychiatrically hospitalized. A study of the Dade County Jail in Miami reported that 10 percent of the prisoners were taking antipsychotic drugs, a number consistent with antipsychotic medication use in many other jails; thus, 10 percent would appear to be a reasonable estimate.[13]

As of mid-2005, a total of 2,186,230 prisoners were incarcerated in local jails and state and federal prisons in the United States. Assuming that 10 percent of them were seriously mentally ill, that would translate into approximately 218,600 seriously mentally ill prisoners. That is more than the entire population of Akron, Ohio; Madison, Wisconsin; Montgomery, Alabama; Richmond, Virginia; or Tacoma, Washington.

Another way to look at the magnitude of the problem is to ascertain the percentage of seriously mentally ill persons who have been arrested. Two large studies carried out by NAMI (the National Alliance for the Mentally Ill) reported that 40 percent (1992 survey) and 44 percent (2003 survey) of seriously mentally ill individuals had been arrested.[14]

Although a debate continues regarding the precise size of the incarceration problem, there is widespread consensus on many other aspects of it. Most observers agree that there are many more mentally ill persons in jails and prisons today than there were in the past. A 1930 study of almost ten thousand arrestees reported that just 1.5 percent of them were psychotic; at that time, most severely mentally ill individuals were in psychiatric hospitals.[15] It is also widely acknowledged that the number of seriously mentally ill persons in jails and prisons has increased sharply in recent years. In the Georgia prison system, for instance, the number of inmates being treated for mental illness increased 73 percent between 1999 and 2006.[16] As a result, jails and prisons have become, de facto, the largest psychiatric institutions in the United States. There are now more mentally ill individuals in the Los Angeles County Jail, Chicago's Cook County Jail, and New York Riker's Island Jail than in any psychiatric hospital in the nation. Despite many inquiries, I have been unable to locate a single county among the 3,139 counties in the

United States in which the local psychiatric unit holds as many seriously mentally ill individuals as the county jail holds on any given day. Jails and prisons have become the nation's primary "hospitals" for the mentally ill.

Jails and prisons were not created to be psychiatric hospitals, and their staffs were not selected or trained to be psychiatric nurses. Some of the problems precipitated by the rise in seriously mentally ill inmates include the following:

- **Suicide:** Multiple studies have reported that at least half of all jail suicides are carried out by individuals who are seriously mentally ill.
- **Abuse and beatings:** These are often the consequence of mentally ill inmates' breaking the rules or physically or verbally assaulting corrections officers. A Department of Justice study reported that mentally ill inmates do these things twice as often as non–mentally ill inmates. Abuse and beatings may also be in response to the disruptive behavior caused by the person's mental illness.
- **Rape:** This occurs commonly. For example, in California, a severely mentally ill man "was in the jail forensic program several times and on two different occasions, he was taken from there and put into a cell with homosexuals who gang raped him."[17]
- **Murder:** In Mississippi, a forty-three-year-old man with paranoid schizophrenia was beaten to death by his eighteen-year-old cellmate, who was being held for armed robbery and murder. In New Jersey, a sixty-five-year-old mentally ill retired stockbroker was raped and stomped to death by his cellmate, who had a history of rape and violence.[18]

"As If He Were a Trained Animal"

In his important book *Crazy*, Pete Earley described Gilbert, an inmate in the Dade County Jail in Miami who was "so mentally impaired that he couldn't speak." He would simply stand naked in his cell, staring out at the corridor. "It was as if the cell's glass front wall that separated him from the rest of the cell block was a television screen and we were moving across it like actors in a confused drama." Although Gilbert had been successfully treated with antipsychotic medication in the past, he could not be involuntarily medicated under Florida law, because he was not considered to be a danger to himself or others. "For two weeks, the only way officers could get Gilbert to obey their commands was by offering him food, as if he were a trained animal, being rewarded with treats."

Pete Earley, **Crazy: A Father's Search through America's Mental Health Madness** *(New York:* **G. P. Putam's Sons, 2006), pp. 86–87.**

Repeat offenders, commonly referred to as "frequent flyers," pose an acute problem for the penal system. A Florida study of such offenders reported that all of them were substance abusers and that half were also mentally ill. Examples include George Wooten in Denver, diagnosed with schizophrenia and substance abuse, who had over 100 bookings, and Gloria Rodgers in Memphis, severely mentally ill, who had 259 arrests for assault, theft, prostitution, public drunkenness, and disturbing the peace. A young Miami man with bipolar disorder was arrested 51 times for minor crimes in one year and 44 times the next year: "One day, he was released from jail and arrested *twenty minutes later* less than one block away."[19]

Mentally ill individuals not only end up in jail more often than non–mentally ill ones, but they also stay longer. A study in Florida reported that mentally ill prisoners stayed, on average, twice as long as other inmates. In Pennsylvania, mentally ill inmates were three times as likely as non–mentally ill prisoners to serve their maximum sentence.[20]

Mentally ill persons are also disproportionately arrested for minor crimes. One study reported that mentally ill jail inmates were "four times more likely to have been incarcerated for less serious charges such as disorderly conduct and threats." Many of these crimes are directly related to the person's untreated illness. For example:

- In New Mexico, a woman with schizophrenia went into a department store and began rearranging the shelves because she had a delusion that she worked there; she was arrested for striking the police officers who asked her to leave.
- In Virginia, a man with schizoaffective disorder was arrested for breaking into a stranger's house and taking a bubble bath.
- In Utah, a mentally ill man was arrested for shoplifting cupcakes; he explained that he was "releasing the Twinkies because they were calling to him."[21]

Given the increasing number of mentally ill individuals in jails and prisons, the impact on the way police and sheriffs in the community do their job has been profound. In New York City in 1976, police took approximately 1,000 mentally ill persons to hospital emergency rooms for evaluation; by 1986, the number had increased to 18,500 and, by 1998, to almost 25,000 per year. The New York Police Department has been called "the world's largest psychiatric outreach team." In suburban Philadelphia, "mental-illness-related incidents" handled by the police more than quadrupled over a four-year period.[22]

- **2006:** In Des Moines, Iowa, police were called to the residence of Joe Martens eighty-eight times between 2000 and 2006. Martens, diagnosed with bipolar disorder, periodically stopped taking his medication, leading to disrupting and threatening behavior. When police respond to calls from his house, "they bring two units; a third helps if things are slow."[23]

The most profound impact mentally ill persons have had on the police and sheriffs has been an increase in the number of the mentally ill killed by law enforcement officers and the number of law enforcement officers killed by the mentally ill. When a law enforcement officer kills someone, it is often classified as a justifiable homicide. The two most common types of justifiable homicides occur when an individual attacks an officer, or when an officer kills an individual who is in the process of committing a crime.

Figure 2.

Justifiable Homicides by Law Enforcement Officers That Were Precipitated by an Attack on the Officer, as a Percentage of All Justifiable Homicides by Law Enforcement Officers for Each Year, 1976–2004

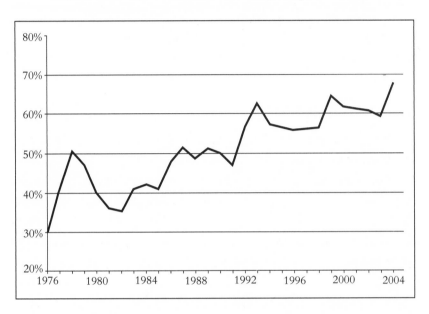

In 2006, the U.S. Department of Justice released data showing that the total number of justifiable homicides had remained relatively constant between 1976 and 2004 but that the *percentage* of such homicides caused by attacks on law enforcement officers had increased sharply. In 1976, for example, attacks on officers accounted for only 30 percent (124 out of 420) of the justifiable homicides; in 2004, however, they accounted for 68 percent (250 out of 368). This increasing percentage of justifiable homicides caused by attacks on law enforcement officers is seen in figure 2.[24]

Data from New York City and Seattle suggest that approximately one-third of the victims of justifiable homicides are mentally ill persons. As was noted in chapter 4, mentally ill individuals accounted for more than half (18 out of 32) of all justifiable homicides by police in

California's Ventura County over a ten-year period.[25] If we extrapolate New York's and Seattle's numbers to a national level and posit that one-third of persons killed by law enforcement officers are people with severe psychiatric disorders, then in 2004 they would have numbered approximately 120. Such homicides are usually provoked by the mentally ill person's attacking the officer. Many officers are poorly trained to handle these crises and shoot to defend themselves or out of fear. With police and sheriffs acting as de facto frontline community mental health workers, encounters between mentally ill persons and officers are on the rise. And, more and more often, the encounters have tragic results.

- **2003, Florida:** Thomas Wallace was killed by police after he attacked an officer. Wallace, who had earned a master's degree in marine biology before becoming afflicted with paranoid schizophrenia, was living in an abandoned water tank and not taking medication.
- **2004, Alabama:** a deputy sheriff killed Annie Holiday, a seventy-eight-year-old woman, after she fired at him. She had been shooting randomly from her house, narrowly missing a young boy. Holiday had paranoid schizophrenia.
- **2004, Indiana:** Kenneth Anderson was killed by police after he killed one officer and wounded five others. Anderson had schizophrenia and was not taking medication.

A substantial but undefined number of these killings are actually planned suicides, commonly referred to as "suicide by cop."

- **2003, Tennessee:** Harold Kilpatrick was killed by police after taking a classroom of students hostage. Kilpatrick had bipolar disorder and was not taking medication. He left a suicide note indicating that he intended to die.
- **2004, North Carolina:** Ronnie Boles was killed by a deputy sheriff after first shooting at the officer. Boles had bipolar disorder and

had planned his death, leaving a note for his family saying, "Everything is going to be over today."

Deaths of law enforcement officers at the hands of mentally ill persons are less common but no less tragic. Although no official organization compiles such data, newspaper accounts collected by the Treatment Advocacy Center suggest that this type of homicide has increased in the last decade, presumably related to the increasing number of seriously mentally ill individuals who are not receiving treatment. For example:

- **2004, Arizona:** Douglas Tatar killed two police officers who came to his apartment to investigate the shooting of another man. Tatar had paranoid schizophrenia; his family had tried to get him committed for treatment two months previously, but the mental health workers said he did not meet the standards for commitment.
- **2004, Alabama:** Clark Barksdale called police and then killed two police officers when they arrived in his driveway. He was diagnosed with schizophrenia and believed that the police were aliens and were sending microwaves into his brain. He had had five previous involuntary commitments but had not been mandated to take medication.

Victimization

The third major consequence of deinstitutionalization and laws making it difficult to treat mentally ill individuals is victimization. People with untreated schizophrenia and bipolar disorder are often confused and disoriented, leaving them vulnerable to those who would rob or rape them. Their judgment is frequently impaired, leading them into dangerous situations. Psychotic behavior, such as manic outbursts or paranoid accusations, may also make them targets of retaliation by others, especially by strangers who are not aware that they are mentally ill.

Despite their many shortcomings, one of the main purposes of psychiatric hospitals was to provide protection for the mentally ill who could not protect themselves. That is why they were called asylums. When released into the community without treatment, many mentally ill individuals are extremely vulnerable. As described by an editorial commenting on the murder of two mentally ill persons, "They are rabbits forced to live in company with dogs."[26]

As deinstitutionalization got underway, there were isolated incidents of mentally ill individuals—usually women who were brutally murdered—whose deaths came to public attention. These incidents occurred relatively seldom in the 1960s and 1970s because, as explained in chapter 1, the patients who were initially discharged from hospitals were those who were least sick and thus least likely to be victimized. However, the early incidents were harbingers of larger things to come:

- In March, 1973, the media in Washington, D.C., reported the murder of Sheila Broughel, an attractive young Phi Beta Kappa graduate of Vassar College who had schizophrenia. Despite multiple brief psychiatric hospitalizations, she had no insight into her illness, refused to take medication voluntarily, and used civil liberties lawyers to defeat all attempts by her family to get her adequately treated. While wandering outside Washington's Union Station, she appeared to be so overtly psychotic and disabled that a *Washington Post* reporter took her to a local psychiatric hospital, where she refused voluntary admission and was assessed as not being sufficiently psychotic to meet the District's strict criteria for involuntary admission. That same night, she was raped and stabbed to death so brutally that her sister could identify her body only "by the teeth." Her sister noted that "she was outwitting whoever was trying to help her. . . . Her rights as a sick person were such that she was able to be prevented from getting the help she needed."[27]
- In April 1981, the media in New York City reported the murder of Phyllis Iannotta, an elderly woman with schizophrenia. She had worked in a factory and helped support her parents for many years

before becoming sick. She was psychiatrically hospitalized but had no awareness of her illness and refused to take medication. At the time of her death, she was living alternately in a public shelter or on a bench in the Port Authority Bus Terminal. She was found in an alley, having been raped and stabbed to death—"her head was bashed in. . . . There was blood everywhere." A shelter operator who knew Ms. Iannotta was asked why they had not had her committed to a hospital. The shelter operator "laughed without a trace of humor. 'Well, she wasn't about to commit herself to a hospital,' she said. 'And the state wouldn't commit her unless she was homicidal or suicidal. That's the law. Phyllis wasn't holding a gun to anybody's head. Simple as that. That's a fact of life around here.'"[28]

By the mid-1980s, reports of similar incidents were proliferating, and initial studies of victimization were being published. In Los Angeles, 278 "psychiatrically disabled" residents of board-and-care homes were interviewed; two-thirds of them "reported having been robbed and/or assaulted during the preceding year." In New York, among twenty women with schizophrenia, half "reported having been raped at least once, with half of these claiming to have been raped more than once."[29]

Throughout the late 1980s and 1990s, increasing data indicated that mentally ill women were especially vulnerable.

- **1987, Virginia:** The "skeletal remains" of Charlotte Powell were found with suggestions that she had been raped and killed. "She had a history of mental problems and was known to wander from home and to hitchhike."
- **1988, Washington, D.C.:** Ella Starks was raped and stabbed, and she "died of asphyxiation when an umbrella was forced down her throat." Severely mentally ill and homeless, she spent her days "waving a large Bible, praying, singing, and sometimes preaching to anyone who cared to listen."

A study of ninety-nine "episodically homeless, seriously mentally ill women" in Washington, D.C., reported that 28 percent of them had been physically assaulted or raped in the preceding month.[30]

Mentally ill men, especially those who were homeless, were also considered easy marks.

- **1989, Des Moines:** Van Mill, suffering from schizophrenia, was robbed and beaten to death by two teenage boys in a public park. The boys tossed Mill "into an empty wading pool at the park and at least one of them jumped up and down on his chest, crushing his small frame."
- **1990, New York:** Thomas Ebbers, a graduate of Brown University but suffering from a "nervous breakdown" and alcoholism, was robbed and stabbed to death.

Most often, people who are mentally ill are victimized by criminals, but occasionally the perpetrators are other mentally ill individuals. In San Francisco, for example, Joshua Rudiger was charged with murder and attempted murder after a series of slashings of homeless persons; Rudiger "told the police that he was a vampire who drank his victims' blood."[31]

In recent years, numerous studies have documented the victimization of the mentally ill. In Pittsburgh, 15 percent of mentally ill individuals living in the community were victims of a violent crime in a ten-week period. Similarly, in Los Angeles, 34 percent were violently victimized over three years. In that study, "a greater severity of clinical symptoms" was the single strongest predictor of victimization, even more so than substance abuse.[32] This relationship between severity of symptoms and likelihood of being victimized was also seen in a Baltimore study of mentally ill women. In short, the sicker people are, the more likely they are to be victimized. The corollary to this fact is that if you treat them and reduce their symptoms, you reduce their chances of being victimized. A North Carolina study of mentally ill individuals for whom treatment was mandated and mentally ill individuals who may or may not have been taking medications showed that the individuals undergoing mandatory treatment were victimized only half as often as those in the other group.[33] In the most useful recent study for quantifying the victimization of individuals with severe mental illnesses, 936 patients living in Chicago were interviewed. During the preceding year, one-quarter of them had been victims of a violent crime. When the results were compared with those of a National Crime Victimization Survey, the mentally ill individuals had been the victims of property theft four times more often than the general population, robbery eight times, assault fifteen times, and rape or attempted rape twenty-two times. The most disturbing aspect of this study was the probability that it underestimated victimization, because the sickest patients refused to participate or were for other reasons not included.[34]

The most troubling form of victimization of mentally ill individuals occurs when their protectors become the perpetrators. The *New York Times* reporter Clifford Levy wrote an astonishing account of this phenomenon in 2002. Levy documented how severely mentally ill residents of group homes in New York were forced to have unnecessary eye operations and prostate surgery in order to generate Medicare fees for unethical physicians and group home operators. In one group home alone, Levy identified over thirty residents who had had unnecessary glaucoma or laser surgery and twenty-four who had had prostate surgery; at least eight residents had undergone both. The eye doctor involved later pled guilty to fraud and billing "for more than 10,000 services that were either improper, unnecessary, or never conducted." Group home operators in other parts of the country have been convicted of stealing funds from their mentally ill residents. In Kansas, the owners of a group home were convicted of "forcing them to work naked" on their farm and "perform sex acts," then billing Medicare for "nude therapy," which they claimed was "beneficial for schizophrenic patients."[35]

9 | The Consequences of Unconstrained Civil Liberties: Violent and Homicidal

> *In this zeal for liberty, many hundreds of sick persons are annually deprived of the liberty of obtaining the medical treatment they require, obtaining in exchange only the liberty to commit suicide or homicide.*

> "LUNATICS AT LARGE AND THE PUBLIC PRESS,"
> *JOURNAL OF MENTAL SCIENCE*, 1898

Among the consequences of failing to treat individuals with severe mental illnesses living in the community, violent behavior and homicides are the most alarming. A cynosure for the media, the stories invariably lead to the stigmatization of mentally ill persons. Day after week after month, reports of such violence offer painful reminders that deinstitutionalization, as carried out in the United States, has for many been a tragic failure.

The incidence of violent behavior among individuals with severe psychiatric disorders can be measured in a number of ways. One approach is to assess violent behavior among those who are psychiatrically hospitalized. Those individuals, however, are not an ideal sample population, since it was often violent behavior that led to their hospitalization. In a North Carolina study of 331 psychiatric inpatients, in the four months preceding admission 51 percent of them had used a weapon to threaten or harm someone or had assaulted someone and caused an injury. Researchers concluded that nonadherence to medication and substance abuse were the main predictors of violent behavior among patients in the study.[1]

Another yardstick for measuring violence involves asking family members about it. In 1992, a large study of over fourteen hundred families was carried out by the National Alliance for the Mentally Ill (NAMI). The families were asked whether their ill family member had physically harmed anyone or threatened to do so in the past year; 11 percent answered that their family member had harmed someone, and an additional 19 percent said their family member had threatened to do so.[2]

A more accurate assessment of violent behavior can be gleaned from systematic studies of mentally ill persons living in the community. In the United States in recent years, there have been eight major studies, summarized in appendix A. It is difficult to compare the results of these studies directly, since the selection of study populations varied from random to highly selective. For example, the CATIE study, funded by the National Institute of Mental Health, included only individuals who were aware of their illness and willing to continue taking antipsychotic medication. Some of the study populations were also biased toward lower rates of violence by the refusal rate of those who were asked, but who refused, to participate in the study, and by the dropout rate during the study.[3] The MacArthur Violence Risk Assessment study had an initial refusal rate of 29 percent (including 44 percent among individuals with schizophrenia) and a study dropout rate of 50 percent.[4] Individuals with paranoid schizophrenia are much less likely, as a result of their suspiciousness, to agree to participate in such studies and are more likely to drop out. They are also known to have high rates of violent behavior.

The results of the studies vary, depending on the diagnoses of the subjects; the percentage of men (who tend to be more violent) included; how violence was defined; how violent behavior was ascertained; the length of time the subjects were followed; and, most important, the number of subjects who were substance abusers and the number who were receiving psychiatric treatment. The CATIE trial included only individuals with schizophrenia and a high percentage (74 percent) of men, but all subjects were being treated with antipsychotic medication. This resulted in a rate of serious violence of only 4 percent in a six-month period.[5] By comparison, treatment of individuals in the Worcester-Philadelphia study was not mandated, resulting in a serious violence rate of 18 percent in a five-month period.[6]

Perhaps the two most troubling studies are the ECA and the MacArthur Violence Risk Assessment studies. The former included a random selection of individuals living in Durham, North Carolina, and Los Angeles; a majority (56 percent) were women; and violence was ascertained by self-report only. Despite these factors, which would tend to produce a low incidence of violent behavior, 7 percent of individuals diagnosed with a major mental disorder who were not also substance abusers and 23 percent who were also substance abusers had used a weapon in a fight or had had more than one physical fight with someone other than a spouse/partner in the preceding year.[7]

The MacArthur study followed 951 individuals discharged from psychiatric hospitals. Despite high refusal and dropout rates, which potentially removed many of the most violent individuals, the 951 individuals committed a total of 608 acts of serious violence (physical injury, threat or assault with a weapon, or sexual assault) in a one-year period. The violence included six homicides and occurred even though mental health authorities contacted these persons every ten weeks during the study period. Overall, 18 percent of the mentally ill persons who were not also substance abusers, and 31 percent who were also substance abusers, committed an act of serious violence.

Although there are fewer European studies that focus on acts of violence other than homicides, those that exist are consistent with the American studies. An English study of 168 individuals with recent-onset psychosis found that 10 percent were seriously violent (used weapon, caused injury, or made a sexual assault) in a three-year period. In another study, of 112 individuals being discharged from an English psychiatric hospital, 19 percent had committed a violent act (physical injury, use of weapon, or sexual assault) within six months. A third English study, of 271 individuals with schizophrenia, reported that 25 percent of them "physically assaulted another person" in a two-year period, a finding the authors called "alarming."[8]

Another method researchers use to assess violent behavior among mentally ill individuals follows unselected birth cohorts over time. In Sweden, for example, all 15,117 individuals who had been born in Stockholm in 1953 were evaluated through case registries thirty years later to ascertain how many had been diagnosed with a "major mental disorder" ("schizophrenia, major affective disorder, paranoid states, and other psychoses") and had *also* been convicted of a violent crime ("the use or threat of physical violence"). It was found that 15 percent of men and 6 percent of women with a major mental disorder had also been convicted of a violent crime.[9]

Birth cohort studies in Finland and Denmark yielded similar results. Criminal convictions for violent crimes (e.g., assault, robbery, arson, rape, murder) were ascertained for all individuals with psychoses up to age twenty-six (Finland) and all individuals with schizophrenia up to age forty-four (Denmark) from specific birth cohorts. In both studies, 7 percent of the mentally ill individuals had a criminal conviction for a violent crime, and in both studies this rate was more than seven times the rate for the general population.[10] This kind of research is possible only in countries that have centralized case registries for individuals treated for mental illness and for the reporting of crimes. Registries like these are well developed in Scandinavian nations but not in the United States.

What do these studies suggest? *Conservatively, it seems reasonable to predict that 5 to 10 percent of individuals with severe psychiatric disorders will commit acts of serious violence each year.* The percentage will be higher if large numbers of individuals are abusing alcohol or drugs, and also if they are not receiving treatment. The effect of treatment is especially well illustrated by the comparatively low rate of serious violence in the CATIE study. In chapter 10, we'll discuss at greater length the MacArthur study's findings on the importance of treatment in reducing violence.

Homicides

Of all types of violent behavior, homicides are the most carefully documented and—as supreme acts of violence—are widely regarded as a barometer for all violent crimes.

American studies are sparse on homicides committed by mentally ill individuals. The most important was a 1977 study of homicides in Albany County, New York, in which the number of homicides committed by mentally ill individuals for the period before wholesale discharges from psychiatric hospitals (1963–69) was compared with the number of homicides after discharges were underway (1970–75). Although the number of homicides by non–mentally ill individuals did not change between the two periods, the number of homicides by seriously mentally ill individuals increased from one (an eighty-two-year-old man with dementia) to eight, all of whom were diagnosed with schizophrenia. These eight individuals were responsible for 29 percent of all homicides in the county during the six-year period. The authors of the study recommended that additional studies be done and concluded that "closer follow-ups of psychotic patients, especially schizophrenics, could do a lot to improve the welfare of the patient and the community."[11]

A 1985 study assessed all homicides for 1978–80 in California's Contra Costa County, a wealthy county with a comparatively low murder rate. Among the seventy-one convicted homicide offenders, seven (10 percent) were diagnosed with schizophrenia and another had a drug-induced psychosis. All had been evaluated psychiatrically prior to the crimes and had refused medication. One example:

- A twenty-five-year-old man shot two friends nonfatally for no apparent reason. He was hospitalized and diagnosed with paranoid schizophrenia. He refused all treatment except psychotherapy, so medications were not given. He was discharged at his own request, because "the hospital did not feel that there were legal grounds to enforce further involuntary confinement." Two weeks later, he killed both his parents "after bursting into their bedroom in the middle of the night to stab and bludgeon them with a baseball bat."[12]

An American study published in 1994 analyzed 2,655 homicides said to be taken from a "representative sample" of thirty-three counties. Information on mental illness was obtained solely from the files of the prosecutors, increasing the likelihood that evidence of a mental illness would have been minimized. Despite this, the study reported that 4.3 percent of the homicide offenders had a "mental illness," not otherwise specified, other than alcohol or drug abuse.[13]

Studies conducted in countries other than the United States shed more light on this issue. In a group of fourteen such studies (see appendix B for complete data), individuals with schizophrenia, delusional disorder, bipolar disorder, or depression with psychotic features committed an average of 9.3 percent (range 5.3 to 17.9 percent) of the homicides. Especially noteworthy were the high frequency of substance abuse and the low frequency of treatment in the mentally ill offenders who committed homicides.

It is difficult to compare these studies with each other since their methodologies differed. It is also important to note that overall homicide rates vary widely among countries and that the United States has one of the highest. As a result, two countries can have a similar incidence of homicide offenders per total number of seriously mentally ill persons, but if other factors have contributed to an unusually high or low *overall homicide rate*, the *percentage* of homicides caused by mentally ill offenders will be skewed. To take an extreme example, Iceland for many years had a very low overall homicide rate, with only forty-seven total homicide offenders reported between 1900 and 1979. However, thirteen of the offenders had schizophrenia, bipolar disorder, or other psychoses, thus accounting for 28 percent of all homicides.[14] By contrast, the United States has a very high homicide rate, so the percentage attributable to individuals with severe psychiatric disorders is comparatively low.

Given the existing data, is it possible to estimate the percentage of homicides for which individuals with serious mental illnesses are responsible? Studies from other countries report an average of approximately 9 percent, but the total U.S. homicide rate is substantially higher than that of other countries, so the *percentage* attributable to mental illness in this country will be lower. *A conservative estimate, based on existing studies, suggests that seriously mentally ill individuals are responsible for at least 5 percent of homicides in the United States.* This translates into 885 homicides among the 16,192 committed in the United States in 2005. In the forty years between 1966, when deinstitutionalization got fully underway, and 2005, there were 759,383 homicides in the United States. If seriously mentally ill individuals were responsible for 5 percent of them, they would total 37,969 homicides.

Rampage Murders

There is one class of homicides for which individuals with severe psychiatric disorders are responsible for a much higher percentage than 5 percent. These are rampage murders in which the person kills several people, usually strangers, at one time. These murders are not related to crimes such as robberies or to domestic disputes.

In a study published in 2000, the *New York Times* examined 100 rampage murders that occurred between 1949 and 1999. In these incidents 425 persons were killed and 510 others injured. The study found that "48 killers had some kind of formal [psychiatric] diagnosis, often schizophrenia. . . . [They] had shown extreme, irrational suspicion and mistrust . . . 20 had been hospitalized for psychiatric problems; 42 had been seen by mental health professionals."[15] The study included examples such as the following:

- **1985:** Sylvia Seegrist, twenty-five, killed three and wounded seven in a shooting spree in a suburban Philadelphia shopping mall. She had been diagnosed with schizophrenia, had been hospitalized twelve times, had previously stabbed a psychologist, and had tried to kill her mother, yet she was receiving no treatment.
- **1999:** Larry Ashbrook, forty-seven, killed seven and wounded seven

in a shooting spree in a church in Fort Worth. For years, he had suffered from untreated paranoid schizophrenia and thought he was being "targeted" by the FBI and other groups. He had even cemented up his toilet to prevent "them" from spying on him.

Although the study used multiple databases to identify all rampage murders within the fifty-year time frame, 90 of the 100 reported incidents occurred between 1980 and 1999. Even within those years, an FBI database indicated that killings with "three or more victims, non-felony or gang[-related], and not family members," increased by 40 percent between the early 1980s and the early 1990s.[16]

Another study of rampage murders in the United States and Canada supports the findings of the *New York Times* study. Among thirty "mass murderers" whose crimes took place between 1949 and 1998, two-thirds appeared to be severely mentally ill. And, as in the *New York Times* study, the majority of cases occurred from 1985 onward.[17]

Press clippings also give a distinct impression that rampage murders have increased in recent years. In Pittsburgh in 2000, there were two such incidents six weeks apart:

- **March 2000:** Ronald Taylor, diagnosed with paranoid schizophrenia and with multiple past psychiatric hospitalizations, killed three strangers and wounded two others in a Burger King and a Mac-Donald's restaurant. Police found a "Satan List" of targets in his apartment.
- **April 2000:** Richard Baumhammers, a lawyer diagnosed with schizophrenia, killed five and wounded two other members of ethnic minority groups.[18]

All previous rampage murders, however, pale in comparison with that carried out by Cho Seung-Hui in April 2007. A twenty-three-year-old senior at Virginia Tech, Cho killed thirty-two students and teachers in a carefully planned attack. He had previously told his roommate that he had a girlfriend who "was a supermodel and traveled through space," that he had a twin brother, and that he had "vacationed in North Carolina with Vladimir Putin, the Russian President." His behavior and writings were so bizarre that students and faculty alike were afraid of him. Following his harassment of two female students in 2005, Cho was court-mandated to be psychiatrically evaluated; he was held overnight in a local hospital but apparently not treated. He was ordered to get treatment as an outpatient but did not do so. The counseling center at Virginia Tech received a copy of his court order mandating treatment, but it apparently did nothing. According to an official investigation, the center did not accept "involuntary or ordered referrals from any source," and even students with schizophrenia were treated only if they requested it. The Virginia state law for involuntary psychiatric commitment and treatment requires that the person be an "imminent danger" to himself or others or be "substantially unable to care for himself." This is one of the most stringent state commitment statutes in the United States and another example of how changes in mental illness laws in the 1970s and 1980s continue to have real consequences.

After the fact, it became abundantly clear that Cho was, and had for some time been, psychotic. In a paranoid, thought-disordered video that Cho left, he ranted about the wrongs that had been done to him: "You have vandalized my heart, raped my soul and torched my conscience. . . . Jesus loved crucifying me. He loved inducing cancer in my head, terrorizing my heart, and ripping my soul all this time."[19] Thirty-two families were left to mourn and to wonder what went wrong.

Family Members as Targets

Unlike Cho Seung-Hui, most severely mentally ill individuals who become violent do not select their victims at random. Multiple studies have confirmed that "between 50 and 60 percent of the victims are family members"; by contrast, among homicides committed by non–mentally ill individuals, only 16 percent of the victims were family members.[20] Given the frequency of violent behavior among the severely mentally ill, such behavior directed at family members is not uncommon, especially among individuals who are not receiving treatment. In a California study, for example, 11 percent of families reported that their mentally ill family member had physically assaulted other family members in the two weeks preceding hospital admission.[21]

The effects of this violence on family members are usually not publicly discussed and only rarely become apparent. Headlines such as "Couple Lives in Fear of Schizophrenic Son's Return," "Families Under Siege: A Mental Health Crisis," and "My Brother Might Kill Me" hint at what has been called "a national tragedy . . . terrorism in our homes."[22] When the families do speak, their stories are often chilling:

- A thirty-four-year-old man with untreated paranoid schizophrenia lived with his mother. "He heard spirits talking to him. . . . He sat on the living room sofa with a knife at his side. . . . For one entire winter she [his mother] half-slept in her lemon yellow chair by the fireplace, house keys pocketed, the better to escape out the front door if she had to. . . . One night, terrified by his behavior, she climbed out of the second floor window onto the roof, 'cowering behind the chimney.' . . . 'I know he's my son and I love him, but it was unbearable,' she said, her voice quavering. 'He would look at me and it would frighten me. I don't think he knew I was his mother. He would think, maybe, that I was the evil one.'"[23]
- "The thought of being attacked and physically harmed by another is frightening in itself, but when the attacker is your own flesh and blood, it is additional, unspeakable trauma upon trauma as your whole being sways between love and fear. "If a stranger were to be the attacker, you would automatically try to defend yourself, but when it is the one you love, you only try to run because your love would bind your hands."[24]

These families' fear is not unfounded, especially not for mothers. According to one study of homicides committed by mentally ill offenders, "mothers represented the largest single group to be targets for violence." In two studies of mothers who were killed by their children, more than three-quarters of the offenders were severely mentally ill, leading one researcher to conclude that "matricide is the schizophrenic crime." Another study of family homicides reported that the mentally ill person tends to be sicker and to have become ill at a younger age than mentally ill persons who attack other people.[25]

- **1990, Los Angeles, Ca.:** Betty Madeira, suffering from untreated schizophrenia and accompanied by her eleven-year-old son disguised as a girl, stabbed and shot to death her seventy-eight-year-old mother. Madeira believed her mother had "killed nine people and buried their bodies in the desert." Madeira's family had been trying unsuccessfully to get her into psychiatric treatment for two years.
- **1998, Reston, Va.:** Alfred Head, diagnosed with schizophrenia, drove his car into the front door of his mother's house, then beat her to death. His mother had been trying in vain to get treatment for him, even telling one psychiatrist, "What do I have to do, have him kill someone to get him treatment?"
- **2006, Caratunk, Me.:** William Bruce, diagnosed with schizophrenia, bludgeoned his mother and then cut her throat. Bruce had been hospitalized but refused to take his medication. According to a friend of the mother's, "She tried to get help everywhere. At each phase she was turned away because he never hurt anyone."[26]

Fathers are victims of violence less frequently than mothers. One study suggested that two-thirds of sons charged with killing their fathers or stepfathers were seriously mentally ill.

- **1985, Nicholasville, Ky.:** James Rankin, diagnosed with schizophrenia, killed his stepfather with a high-power bow and arrow. He had been hospitalized three times the preceding year, but after each hospitalization he stopped taking his medication and became increasingly paranoid.
- **1997, Indianapolis, Ind.:** James Garner, diagnosed with schizophrenia, stabbed his father to death, dismembered the body, and ate

part of the brain. He believed that "his father was the devil and killed him to release spirits from his body."[27]

The murder of parents or other family members by a son or daughter is uncommon but not rare. In California in 2005, there were thirty such murders. However, in 2007 in Contra Costa County, with a population of approximately one million, three such murders occurred in a four-month period. The perpetrators were described as having schizophrenia and not taking his medication; having "emotional problems and not taking his medication"; and having "a history of mental illness."[28]

The most highly publicized form of violence against family members is violence against children. Child murders (filicide) committed by mentally ill mothers or fathers attract much public attention, witness the 2001 case of Andrea Yates in Houston. Yates, who had been hospitalized multiple times for severe depression and psychosis, drowned her five children on instructions from Satan.

Few systematic studies of child murders have been done. A review of cases published in 1969, before most patients had been released from psychiatric hospitals, reported that 21 percent of the parents were "acutely psychotic." A more recent review (2005) separated mothers who killed their children on the day they were born (neonaticide) from those who killed their children later. Many women in the neonaticide group were "young, poor, [and] unmarried," whereas "approximately one-half of the mothers" in the latter group had psychosis or severe depression. A similar study in Sweden reported that two-thirds of parents who killed their children had "some kind of mental illness."[29]

Some media coverage of the Andrea Yates case implied that such killings are rare events. In fact, when Yates went to prison in 2002 she joined sixty-nine other women serving time in the Texas prison system for killing one or more of their children.[30] In one seven-month period in 2003, four filicide incidents were reported in Texas alone:

- **March 2003, Brownsville:** John Rubio, diagnosed with paranoid schizophrenia, killed his own child and two others, ages two months and three years, because he believed they were "possessed by demons."

- **May 2003, Tyler:** Deanna Laney, who had had psychotic episodes for at least three years but had not been treated, beat to death her six- and eight-year-old sons and severely injured her fourteen-month-old son. She said she was carrying out God's orders.

- **September 2003, Houston:** Demetria Evans, who had a history of severe depression and violent behavior but was not taking her medication, killed her nine-year-old daughter by strangulation.

- **September 2003, Plano:** Lisa Diaz, suffering from schizophrenia, drowned her two daughters, ages three and five. Three weeks earlier, she had been referred to a psychiatrist.

During this same seven-month period, many similar incidents were reported in other states:

- **July 2003, Minneapolis:** Naomi Gaines, diagnosed with severe depression with psychotic features, threw her fourteen-month-old twin boys from a bridge into the Mississippi River, killing one of them. Gaines was well known to local police and child protection workers because of her previous erratic behavior.

- **September 2003, Las Vegas:** Sylvia Ewing, suffering from severe depression, beat to death her children, ages four and eight. She had been evaluated and given medication, but it is not known whether she was taking it.

Invariably, these cases feature a lack of current psychiatric treatment, although most of the women had received previous treatment. A recent study of women in the United States who had killed their children found that three-quarters of them had received prior psychiatric care, and half of them had been previously psychiatrically hospitalized.[31]

Public Figures as Targets

In episodes of violence committed by individuals with serious psychiatric disorders, a significant number of the victims are public figures. Entertainers are frequently targeted, witness the attacks on John Lennon, shot to death in 1980 by Mark David Chapman, diagnosed with psychosis, and on George Harrison, who was stabbed but not killed in 1999 by a man with paranoid schizophrenia. The stalking of the actress Jodie Foster by John Hinckley is another well-known example. Hinckley, suffering from schizophrenia, attempted to impress Foster in 1981 by shooting President Ronald Reagan.

In addition to acts of violence, mentally ill persons may frighten entertainers by stalking and/or threatening them. Margaret Ray, diagnosed with schizophrenia but usually not on medication, stalked David Letterman for a decade, breaking into his home four times and even stealing his car. Ray believed that she was Letterman's wife; she finally committed suicide in 1998.[32] Studies of people who stalk other people suggest that approximately one-third of them have a serious psychiatric disorder and almost all are not being treated.[33] Some, like Margaret Ray, are relatively harmless. Others, like John Hinckley, are not.

In addition to national figures like David Letterman, local radio and television personalities may be stalked, threatened, or even killed by seriously mentally ill individuals. This is unsurprising, given that many individuals with paranoid schizophrenia believe that people on the radio and/or television are talking about them or sending voices into their head. A 1999 survey of radio and television stations, in which I took part, found that 48 percent of the stations responding to the survey reported having received a call, letter, fax, or email demanding that the station stop talking about them or sending voices to their head. Moreover, 18 percent of the stations had received threats.[34] These sometimes lead to tragic outcomes:

- **1994:** William Tager shot to death an NBC studio employee at the network's New York studio. Tager said that the network had been sending rays through his television set and spying on him for twenty years, "and he couldn't take it anymore."[35]

• **1999:** Lisa Duy, diagnosed with paranoid schizophrenia, shot to death one employee and wounded another employee of a television station in Salt Lake City. Duy claimed that the station was harassing her and putting voices in her head. Three years previously, she had taken a butcher knife to another station and demanded to see a disc jockey. She was ordered to receive psychiatric treatment, but the order expired, and she refused further treatment.[36]

Mentally ill persons sometimes target politicians. At St. Elizabeths Hospital in Washington, D.C., a constant stream of mentally ill persons are admitted after showing up at the White House gate and arguing that they have to see the president to convey to him some secret information. These individuals are known as "White House cases"; a study of 192 of them who were mentally ill reported that they had a significant excess of arrests for violent as well as nonviolent crimes.[37]

Although no formal studies have been done on the phenomenon, religious leaders are commonly targeted by individuals with severe psychiatric disorders. Presumably, they are viewed as representatives of God and become linked to the religious delusions so commonly found in individuals with psychosis, as the cases of Herbert Mullin and Bryan Stanley attest.

Another tragic example of religious leaders as targets occurred in Waterville, Maine, in January 1996. Mark Bechard, diagnosed with schizophrenia and with nine past psychiatric admissions, stabbed and bludgeoned to death two elderly nuns and seriously wounded two others. When he was finally stopped by police officers, Bechard was said to be "standing over one bloodied nun with the statue of the Blessed Mary in his hand."[38] Bechard was known to respond well when he took medication but frequently refused to do so. On the day of the attack, his parents had called the local mental health center, but no weekend staff was available and the crisis line was malfunctioning. Ironically, Bechard had previously been included in a class action suit against a Maine state psychiatric hospital, which led to the release of many patients and made it more difficult to hospitalize people like himself.

The media regularly report homicides in which religious figures are the victims:

- **1999, Connecticut:** Michael Ouellette, diagnosed with schizophrenia and with two previous psychiatric hospitalizations, beat to death a Catholic priest with a candle stand.[39]
- **2002, New York:** Peter Troy, with a thirteen-year history of paranoid schizophrenia and multiple hospitalizations, shot to death a Catholic priest as he was performing morning Mass and also killed an elderly parishioner. According to a newspaper account, after an earlier discharge from a psychiatric hospital, "county mental health caseworkers were supposed to check on him," but "they lost track and improperly closed his record."[40]

Mental Health Professionals

Perhaps unsurprisingly, mental health professionals also appear to be a common target for individuals with severe psychiatric disorders. According to data compiled by the U.S. Department of Justice, the annual rate of job-related victimization by violent crime was 12.6 incidents per 1,000 workers. For physicians, the rate was 16.2 per 1,000, but for psychiatrists and other mental health professionals the rate was 68.2 per 1,000, more than five times the average. This high rate is confirmed by state statistics. In Washington State, workers at psychiatric hospitals have the highest rate of any group for violence-related injuries, a rate eight times higher than that of police officers.[41]

Simple assault by severely mentally ill individuals against mental health professionals is relatively common, especially in psychiatric hospitals that serve psychotic patients. Surveys of psychiatrists suggest that between one-third and one-half of them have experienced at least one assault.[42] Sometimes the assault occurs after the patient has been discharged.

- **1998, California:** Kathryn Schoonover, who was severely mentally ill, was arrested for sending a package of potassium cyanide to a nurse in the hospital where she had been a patient. Schoonover had a "hit list" containing the names of other hospital employees.[43]

Psychiatrists appear to be the most likely to be involved in fatal episodes. In separate cases in Oregon in 1985, severely mentally ill patients killed two psychiatrists in a five-month period. There is no central registry for homicides like these, but they occur sporadically.

- **2006, Maryland:** Vitali Davydov, diagnosed with schizophrenia, beat to death his psychiatrist, Dr. Wayne Fenton, who was a prominent expert on this disorder. Davydov had been off medication for two months and hallucinated that Fenton had asked to be killed because he "wanted his soul to leave his body."[44]

Psychiatric nurses, social workers, and outreach workers making home visits to patients in the community are also vulnerable, since they do not have any backup assistance if patients become agitated:

- **1999, New York:** Diane Wylie, seriously mentally ill, bludgeoned to death a psychiatric nurse who was making a home visit to see how Wylie was doing.
- **2005, Washington, D.C.:** Larry Clark, diagnosed with schizophrenia and not taking his medication, stabbed to death a mental health worker who had been summoned to the house by Clark's mother.

As increasing numbers of severely ill patients are moved from hospitals to community residences and receive inadequate treatment, the number of such tragedies is likely to increase.[45]

Repeat Offenders

The single most important predictor of violent behavior is a history of violent behavior. This is true for people who are not mentally ill and even more so for people who are. A Finnish study of individuals who had committed two homicides several years apart (homicide recidivists) reported that being a male increased the odds of homicide recidivism ten times, and alcoholism increased it thirteen times, but having schizophrenia increased it more than twenty-five times.[46]

It is therefore inexplicable why so many severely mentally ill individuals with a documented history of violent behavior are being released with no follow-up psychiatric care. Two decades ago, the psychiatrist Richard Lamb detailed the magnitude of the problem. A two-year follow-up study of severely mentally ill individuals who had been arrested for felony crimes in Los Angeles revealed the following: one-third (8 out of 24) of the "psychotic habitual criminal" group and more than one-half (7 out of 13) of the "frequently violent psychotic" group had been released from jail "with no provision for postrelease treatment." As Lamb noted, "Simply to release these seriously mentally ill persons who have, in addition, high proved potential for antisocial and violent acts does a tremendous disservice to these patients as well as to society. . . . These mentally ill persons cry out for treatment and social controls and their cries should not go unheard."[47]

As we have sown, so we have reaped. The following are examples of recidivist homicides by mentally ill individuals in the 1990s:

- **1993, Virginia:** Jeanette Harper, diagnosed with bipolar disorder, stabbed to death an elderly woman who had taken Harper in as a houseguest. Seven years before, Harper had shot to death a black man because she believed he was conspiring to murder her; she was hospitalized for two years, then released. Harper had been evaluated by the local mental health center multiple times prior to the second murder, including just one hour earlier, but the center had said she did not meet criteria for involuntary commitment. Harper was said to respond well to medication but had stopped taking it.

- **1999, Michigan:** Paul Harrington, diagnosed with depression with psychosis, killed his wife and son. Twenty-four years earlier, Harrington, in a virtually identical crime, had killed his first wife and two daughters; he was hospitalized for two months and released. Prior to the second murders, he had run out of the medication he took to control his depression and voices.

- **1999, New York:** Salvatore Grassi, diagnosed with schizophrenia, killed his wife, who was trying to get psychiatric care for him. According to an account of the murder, "The day before he killed her, she was on the phone for quite some time. . . . It seemed like getting help was just impossible." Sixteen years earlier, Grassi had shot to death their son and was subsequently hospitalized for eight years. Prior to both homicides, Grassi had stopped taking his medication.[48]

The Extraordinary Case of Dr. John Kappler

As exhibit A to illustrate the failure of the psychiatric profession to treat mentally ill individuals who have proven dangerous, John Kappler probably has no peer. A physician who practiced anesthesiology, Kappler also had bipolar disorder with psychosis (auditory hallucinations) and antisocial (sociopathic) personality traits. Apparently responding to voices, he unsuccessfully attempted to kill three patients in 1975, causing brain damage to one of them. In 1980, he tried to kill another patient, and in 1985, he turned off the respirator on another; both patients were revived, but there are indications that Kappler may have succeeded in killing others. Despite these incidents, he continued to practice medicine during this ten-year period, the cover-up by his family and friends matched only by the incompetence of his treating psychiatrist. Even though he responded very well to antipsychotic medications during hospitalizations, at no time was he mandated to continue taking them. Finally, in 1990 Kappler ran his car over and killed a random bicyclist, who also turned out to be a physician, and severely wounded a woman. At this point, he was convicted of homicide and sent to prison.

The story is told by Keith Ablow in The Strange Case of Dr. Kappler: The Doctor Who Became a Killer (New York: Free Press, 1994).

In other cases, the homicide by the mentally ill person was preceded by other crimes that should have led to ongoing treatment:

- **1998, Iowa:** Daniel Ellis, diagnosed with bipolar disorder, drove through a stop sign at seventy miles per hour, killing an elderly man. Five years earlier, Ellis had been charged with attempted murder when he grabbed a three-year-old boy in a park and jumped into the Des Moines River. At that time, a judge ordered Ellis's psychiatrist to report monthly on whether Ellis was taking his medication, but the reports were not sent. Ellis had been off medication for two weeks at the time of the homicide.[49]

The release of such individuals without ensuring follow-up treatment simply defies common sense.

Summary: The Consequences of Unconstrained Civil Liberties

For almost half a century, we have released seriously mentally ill persons into the community but failed to treat them. The consequences include the following:

1. A massive increase in seriously mentally ill persons who are homeless. They number approximately 175,000 and constitute at least one-third of the total homeless population. When they are untreated, the incidence of violent crime among such individuals is forty times higher than that among those who are being treated.

2. A massive increase in seriously mentally ill persons in jails and prisons. They number approximately 218,600 and constitute at least 10 percent of the jail and prison population. There are now more seriously mentally ill individuals in county jails than in any county psychiatric facility, and jails have become America's primary mental hospitals.

3. Police and sheriffs have become the nation's frontline mental health workers. Increasing confrontations between law enforcement officials and mentally ill persons are ending tragically for one or the other; at least one-third of the victims of justifiable homicides by police and sheriffs are individuals with serious psychiatric disorders.

4. Victimization of seriously mentally ill individuals living in the community has become a fact of life. Approximately one-quarter of them are victims of violent crime each year, and one-third of the women have been raped.

5. Between 5 and 10 percent of seriously mentally ill persons living in the community will commit a violent act each year, almost all because they are not receiving treatment. In the United States, they are responsible for at least 5 percent of all homicides. Family members are a common target, especially mothers and children. Law enforcement officers, media personalities, politicians, religious leaders, and mental health professionals are also common targets.

10 | An Imperative for Change

The right to treatment is more fundamental than unrestricted liberty. If we do not provide adequate treatment, we offer the patient no freedom at all.

In retrospect, a social disaster was virtually guaranteed when hundreds of thousands of individuals with severe psychiatric disorders were discharged to live in the community without any assurance that they would receive treatment. The dimensions of this disaster are now clear—homelessness, incarceration, victimization, and violent behavior, including homicide. Most of these problems, as noted previously, are associated with a subset of individuals who are unaware of their illness, do not take medication, and/or abuse alcohol and drugs. These individuals are responsible for most episodes of incarceration and violent behavior. According to the Duke University researcher Jeffrey Swanson and his colleagues, this is the "small subset of SMI [seriously mentally ill] individuals, in which the combination of substance abuse and nonadherence to treatment leads to aggressive or threatening behavior."[1]

The first step toward fixing the problem lies in understanding its dimensions. The remedy will not come easily, but continuing on our present course is not acceptable. We must embark on a new course to protect those afflicted, decrease stigma, protect the public, prevent the problem from becoming worse, and make better use of public funds.

Protecting Those Afflicted

The single most compelling reason for correcting the present system of nontreatment is simply that it is the right thing to do. This idea was clearly articulated by Stephen Rachlin, a psychiatrist at the Bronx Psychiatric Center, and his colleagues three decades ago:

> *The humane approach to serious impairment of mental functioning demands that the suffering of the patient be relieved. He must be helped to take his place in society comfortably. We believe that this right is more fundamental than, and therefore takes precedence over, that of liberty, for without appropriate therapy what do we offer the patient? It is true that he is free to come and go as he pleases, but what about the quality of his life? Can we really call it "liberty" if someone walks the streets in terror because of paranoid delusions or threatening hallucinations?*[2]

What kind of civilization allows seriously mentally ill persons to be victimized—to live on the streets and beneath bridges; to be robbed, raped, or even killed; to live in rundown inner-city neighborhoods as easy prey for petty criminals; or to live in unmonitored group homes where they may even be subjected to unnecessary surgery to satisfy someone's greed? A civilization that allows such things cannot claim to be humane.

Mentally ill individuals who end up in jail or prison often suffer needlessly, unable to comprehend the institution's rules. Occasionally, they are incarcerated for long periods for crimes committed as a direct consequence of their untreated mental illness. Many of these individuals rotate between the street and jail, punctuated by brief stays on a psychiatric ward from which they are released to resume their medieval pilgrimage. The Wisconsin psychiatrist Darold Treffert has aptly said that rather than protecting these people's legal rights, we are merely endorsing some "legal rites."[3]

My Brother Sits

Sometimes, late at night, my brother sits in his darkened room watching television without any sound and laughing hysterically. His giggling is punctuated by one-sided, incoherent conversations that he holds with the voices he hears in his head. Doug is 30 years old, and for the past 10 years, he has suffered from schizophrenia, a fact which he neither acknowledges nor accepts. . . . Doug, like many other people who have schizophrenia, cannot or will not realize that something is wrong, and he refuses to take any medication. So for my family, it all becomes useless, all the groundbreaking research and fancy new drugs, because he will not help himself. Sometimes I want to just shake him and scream, "Don't you know? You don't have to be like this!" He is so lonely, so profoundly isolated from all that exists outside the cacophony in his skull. He has no friends, almost no human connection with anyone at all. . . . And there is nothing we can do about it—we have no way to force him to get help. If a person with schizophrenia refuses to take medication, the only recourse is to have him or her involuntarily committed. But you can only do that by proving the person is a danger to him or herself or others. . . . [The] civil libertarians . . . would call this a victory, that a person has some right to be insane. I call it cruel and an enormous waste of human potential.

Jenna Ward, Treatment Advocacy Center website, www.psychlaws.org.

Imagine what would happen today if we treated individuals with severe mental retardation or Alzheimer's disease the same way we treat individuals with severe psychiatric disorders. The public would call it uncivilized and would demand change. And yet this uncivilized treatment is now the norm for those whom John Locke, in 1690, called

"Madmen, which for the present cannot possibly have the use of right Reason to guide themselves." Locke added that protecting such individuals "seems no more than Duty, which God and nature has laid on Man."[4]

Decreasing Stigma

Of all the burdens borne by mentally ill individuals, stigma is one of the heaviest. It affects opportunities for employment, housing, and social relations and becomes a scarlet letter that all mentally ill persons must carry.

The most important cause of stigma against mentally ill persons is episodes of violent behavior by the small subset of patients previously described. However, all mentally ill individuals are being stigmatized because of the behavior of a few. Multiple surveys have noted that the public associates mental illness with violence and that this association is the main source of stigma. In one survey, 38 percent of adults agreed that "people with mental illness are more dangerous than the rest of society." In another, "a majority" of adults said that people with schizophrenia were more likely than other people to commit violent crimes.[5]

In the last two decades, numerous public education campaigns have emphasized that "mentally ill persons make good neighbors." Prominent personalities including Mike Wallace and Patty Duke have publicly discussed their own mental illnesses in an effort to decrease stigma. Americans in general now have a much better understanding of the biological causes of mental illnesses. They have experienced more psychotherapy and had more contact with mental health professionals. Compared with attitudes in decades past, these factors should have led to a marked decrease in stigma against mentally ill persons.

A definitive test of whether that stigma has, in fact, decreased took place in 1996. As part of a national survey, researchers asked a question identical to one that had been asked in a similar survey in 1950: "When you hear someone say that a person is 'mentally ill,' what does that mean to you?" In 1950, 13 percent of respondents included violent behavior in their description of "mentally ill." However, in 1996, *31 percent of respondents* did so. As summarized by the researchers,

> *Perceptions that such people are dangerous increased nearly two and a half times since 1950 to a point that, in 1996, nearly one-third of respondents spontaneously volunteered the idea that psychotic persons may be violent. . . . [S]omething has occurred in our culture over the past half century that has increased the connection between psychosis and violence in the public mind. Whatever that something is, it has had this effect despite our best efforts to achieve exactly the opposite result.*[6]

That "something" is self-evident: the public now perceives mentally ill persons to be more violent because they *are* more violent. The increase in homicides and other violent acts, many of which have been widely publicized, has had exactly the stigmatizing effect that one would predict. As the sociologist Bruce Link and his colleagues put it, "The finding that individuals who believe that mental patients and former mental patients are dangerous . . . can be interpreted relatively straightforwardly. Such individuals find former patients threatening and prefer to maintain a safe social distance from them."[7]

It seems clear that we will never successfully reduce stigma against mentally ill persons until we reduce violent behavior by the subgroup responsible for it. Richard Lamb has noted, "We can reduce stigma by doing what needs to be done to ensure that persons with severe mental illness who resist treatment receive the treatment they so clearly need."[8] Currently, we have a situation where commuters on buses and subways may look up and see a public service ad proclaiming that "mentally ill persons make good neighbors," then look down at their newspaper and read a story about another act of violence by a severely mentally ill person. To try to control stigma without addressing the problem of violence is as futile as trying to control a hurricane without addressing the problem of wind.

Protecting the Public

The present system of psychiatric care needs to be fixed in order to protect the public, since a major function of government is to provide a safe environment for its citizens. With regard to potentially dangerous medical conditions, we have laws prohibiting people with typhoid fever from working in restaurants, we do not allow people with active tuberculosis to use public transportation, and we insist that people with epilepsy take medication if they are going to drive vehicles. In each case, the purpose of the law is to protect the general public from individuals who are potentially dangerous.

Similarly, we should protect the public from that group of individuals with severe psychiatric disorders who are known to be potentially dangerous. It is clear that severely mentally ill individuals are responsible, by conservative estimates, for at least 5 percent of all homicides in the United States and for up to half of all "rampage" murders. Must we wait until such violence increases before we act? Family members, law enforcement officers, media personalities, religious leaders, and mental health professionals are all frequent victims. By not affording protection to these individuals, we are depriving them of *their* civil liberties and sometimes their lives.

Preventing the Problem from Becoming Worse

We must correct our present failure to treat individuals with severe mental illnesses because the problem is growing. The increasing number of mentally ill individuals among the homeless, the increasing number in jails and prisons, and the proliferating reports of victimization all support this conclusion. The increase is most firmly established, however, for episodes of violence, including homicides.

It is instructive to compare the number of homicides committed by mentally ill individuals prior to the beginning of deinstitutionalization with the number in recent years. At least five studies were carried out in the United States between 1900 and 1950, during which time most people with severe psychiatric disorders were confined to state mental hospitals. The percentage of homicide offenders found to be "insane" or "psychotic" in these studies ranged from 1.7 percent to 3.6 percent. In reviewing these studies, the criminologist Marvin Wolfgang concluded that "if the universe from which the insane proportion is taken refers to all those arrested for criminal homicide, the proportion [of those who are severely mentally ill] is usually 2 percent or less."[9] This contrasts with a minimum of 5 percent today.

There are many indicators that violent behavior and homicides committed by seriously mentally ill individuals are a growing problem. A study comparing violent behavior in patients admitted to a New York psychiatric hospital in the early 1980s and the early 1990s reported that "the rates of violence have increased roughly 40 percent for men and 150 percent for women." A study of "mentally disordered offenders who push or attempt to push victims onto subway tracks" in New York City found that the frequency of the offense increased more than twice as fast between 1986 and 1991 than between 1975 and 1985. A study of "rampage" killers in the United States reported a 46 percent increase in such tragedies in 1990–97 compared with 1976–89. Anecdotal accounts of mentally ill individuals attacking family members have also become more numerous. In California, for example, the following report was published in 2001: "In San Bernardino County, prosecutors see more than two new cases a month of adult mentally ill children attacking their parents. . . . Last month [Deputy District Attorney] Svare had five such cases. . . . This type of elder abuse has not been common in the past."[10]

Making Better Use of Public Expenditures

The last reason to change our system of care for individuals with severe psychiatric disorders is that the present system wastes resources. Two studies carried out by the National Institute of Mental Health in the 1990s established the fact that the care of such patients is extremely expensive. In these studies, "severe mental disorders" included individuals with schizophrenia, bipolar disorder, autism, and severe forms of depression, panic disorder, and obsessive-compulsive disorder. In one study, they constituted 13 percent of all individuals with mental disorders yet accounted for 40 percent of the total costs. In the other study, this group accounted for 58 percent of all mental illness treatment costs. In the latter study, the cost of treating an individual in the "severe and persistent" group was estimated to be $19,900 per year, compared with $1,700 per year for an individual with a less severe form of mental illness.[11]

It is therefore apparent that the sickest mental patients account for a large share of the total costs. Moreover, there are suggestions that a subset of the sickest patients—the sickest of the sickest—are especially expensive. In an English study of persons with schizophrenia, the 10 percent of patients with the most severe symptoms accounted for 80 percent of the total costs.[12] If we are ever going to get control of treatment costs for mental illnesses in general, we will have to focus our efforts on the sickest subset.

There is also evidence that costs for treating individuals with severe psychiatric disorders have increased sharply in recent years and are almost certainly still increasing. Most such individuals are supported by federal funds under the Medicaid, Medicare, Supplemental Security Income (SSI), and Social Security Disability Insurance (SSDI) programs. According to numbers provided by the Social Security Administration (but not adjusted for inflation), these costs have risen as follows:

- Medicaid expenditures for mental illnesses almost tripled between 1987 and 1997, from $5.7 billion to $14.4 billion.
- Medicare expenditures for mental illnesses tripled between 1987 and 1997, from $3.0 billion to $9.1 billion.
- Supplemental Security Income (SSI) expenditures for "mental disorders not including mental retardation" more than quadrupled between 1986 and 1998, from $1.5 billion to $7.4 billion.
- Social Security Disability Insurance (SSDI) expenditures for "men-

tal disorders not including mental retardation" more than tripled between 1986 and 1998, from \$3.1 billion to \$11.0 billion.

The total increase in these four programs between 1986–87 and 1997–98 was \$2.6 billion per year, making them among the most rapidly growing programs in the federal budget.[13]

Where does all this money go? Much of it is wasted on repeated psychiatric hospital admissions caused by patients who have limited insight and do not take medication once they are discharged. Studies have shown that noncompliance with medication and substance abuse are the two "most important factors related to frequency of hospitalization."[14]

The frequency of psychiatric readmissions for some individuals is astounding, especially given the reality that readmissions have become increasingly difficult to achieve. In New York State, 40 percent of discharged mentally ill patients are rehospitalized within six months; in Illinois, 30 percent are rehospitalized within one month. One study looked at patients who had had the most lifetime admissions to state psychiatric hospitals: California, Illinois, Oregon, and Texas had patients with more than 60 admissions; Georgia, Massachusetts, and North Carolina had patients with more than 80 admissions; New York had a patient with 98 admissions, and Connecticut had one with 121 admissions. Recent data from Florida identified 247 individuals who had been evaluated for involuntary psychiatric hospitalization 10 or more times in a two-year period.[15]

Even when these mentally ill persons are not being hospitalized or otherwise treated, they still cost money. To qualify for federal benefits under SSI, SSDI, Medicaid, and Medicare requires only that the person be examined and certified as having a serious psychiatric disorder; there is no requirement that the person be in a treatment program as a condition for receiving benefits. Although no data are available on this issue, it is likely that many of the most severely mentally ill but untreated individuals are receiving federal benefits under these programs. For example, Russell Weston, diagnosed with schizophrenia, received federal SSI payments of \$579 per month (in 2005 equivalent dollars) *for fourteen years*, totaling almost $100,000, before coming to Washington in July 1998 and killing two police officers as he stormed the U.S. Capitol. During those years, he was treated only for two months during his single, brief hospitalization. Malcoum Tate received federal SSI payments of $579 per month (in 2005 equivalent dollars) *for eleven years*, totaling over $78,000, during the years when he refused to take medication and terrorized his family. The problem of the Russell Westons and Malcoum Tates who are potentially dangerous and receiving public funds but not being treated is seldom publicly discussed.

Severely mentally ill individuals also consume public funds by engaging free legal representation, one of the hallmarks of the American judicial system. Many patients who have anosognosia have used this system to avoid being treated. Such services are state and federally funded under the Legal Services Corporation and the Protection and Advocacy Program. An example of the abuse of such programs involved David Moser, diagnosed with bipolar disorder, who attempted to kill his elderly parents and used government-funded legal representation to avoid being treated. According to one account of his case,

> *He has been provided with an attorney free of charge by the state of Massachusetts on at least a dozen occasions, commanding over his life[time] hundreds of thousands of dollars in legal attention, but he has never once been forced to take any medication for an illness that psychiatrists describe as eminently treatable.*[16]

Mentally ill individuals also utilize public funds in the corrections system. The costs associated with mentally ill inmates in jail are approximately 60 percent higher than the costs of non–mentally ill inmates. In Broward County, Florida, for example, it costs $125 per day versus $78 per day. These costs include medication and extra staffing for required activities, such as suicide checks. The public mental health system provides funding to fewer than half of the nation's jails to cover these costs, leaving county and state departments of correction to absorb the rest. Getting mentally ill persons off the streets and into jail also strains the correctional system's fiscal resources. A study in California estimated that in one year, city police departments in the state spent $445 million "on handling mentally ill offenders," and county sheriffs spent an additional $160 million.[17]

Finally, given the litigious nature of American society, lawsuits are inevitably associated with the failure to treat individuals with severe psychiatric disorders. Although no national database for calculating such costs exists, it is clear that they are both substantial and increasing:

- **1998, Wisconsin:** A jury awarded $5.4 million to Scott Lawson, a mentally ill man who was placed in solitary confinement for more than two months in a county jail.
- **2004, Tennessee:** Monica Johnson sued the Memphis Police Department for $10.5 million; police had killed her husband, diagnosed with bipolar disorder but not taking medication.
- **2006, New Jersey:** The family of Joel Seidel sued Camden County for "millions of dollars." Seidel, diagnosed with bipolar disorder, was stomped to death by his cellmate in the county jail.

State prison systems have been especially hard hit by lawsuits involving care to prisoners with severe psychiatric disorders. Lawsuits are active or have recently been settled in several states, including Massachusetts, Connecticut, Ohio, Michigan, Wisconsin, Texas, and New Mexico.[18]

Resistance to Dealing with the Problem

Protecting those afflicted, decreasing stigma, protecting the public, preventing the problem from becoming worse, and making better use of public expenditures—these would all seem to be compelling reasons to improve our present system for treating severely mentally ill individuals.

Most of the general public would agree, but for mental health professionals and advocates it is anything but a given. There is a strong aversion among them to acknowledging that some individuals with psychiatric disorders may be dangerous. This aversion dates from the earliest years of the last century, when *The Maniac Barber* (1902) and *The*

Maniac Cook (1909) popularized the image of the homicidal madman. This was followed by such films as *Psycho* (1960) and *Halloween* (1978) and, more recently, the *Friday the 13th* and *Nightmare on Elm Street* series. Among mental health professionals and advocates, it is politically incorrect to acknowledge publicly that mentally ill persons may be dangerous. "The mentally ill are not more dangerous than the general public" is virtually a mantra.

To understand professional resistance to dealing with the issue of violence, it is instructive to examine the work of two prominent researchers, John Monahan, a psychologist, and Henry Steadman, a sociologist. In a joint 1983 publication, Monahan and Steadman claimed that any association between mental illness and violent behavior was a statistical artifact and disappeared when the data were corrected for age, social class, and other demographic variables: "Put another way, the correlates of crime among the mentally ill appear to be the same as the correlates of crime among any other group. . . . [T]here is no relation between crime and mental disorder in the aggregate."[19]

As evidence accumulated in the late 1980s that violent behavior was indeed related to mental illness, this assertion became increasingly untenable. Thus, in 1992, Monahan, commenting on the newly emerging research, noted,

> *The data that have recently become available, fairly read, suggest the one conclusion I did not want to reach: Whether the measure is the prevalence of violence among the disordered or the prevalence of disorder among the violent, whether the sample is people who are selected for treatment as inmates or patients in institutions or people randomly chosen from the open community, and no matter how many social and demographic factors are statistically taken into account, there appears to be a relationship between mental disorder and violent behavior. . . . Denying that mental disorder and violence may be in any way associated is disingenuous and ultimately counterproductive.*[20]

Given statements like this one and the accumulation of additional studies in the 1990s linking violence and mental disorder, one might have predicted that the issue had been settled. Such a prediction would have been mistaken. In 1998, the MacArthur Violence Risk Assessment study discussed in chapter 9 was published, with Monahan and Steadman as authors. It concluded that "there was no significant difference between the prevalence of violence by [mentally ill] patients without symptoms of substance abuse and the prevalence of violence by others living in the same neighborhood who were also without symptoms of substance abuse." A press release issued by Monahan made the point explicit: "Discharged patients who do not abuse alcohol or other drugs are no more violent than their neighbors." The study was widely reported by the media. *Mental Health Weekly* headlined, "Violence Study Dispels Perception of Psychiatric Patients," while the *Washington Post* led with "Are Former Mental Patients More Violent? If They Don't Abuse Drugs or Alcohol, the Answer Is Generally No, Study Finds."[21]

The message was politically correct. According to Monahan, he and the other authors of the study had "conducted focus groups before writing their report" in order to "cast things in the least inflammatory way."[22] Although politically correct, the report reflected only some of the study's findings.

The MacArthur study had followed 951 psychiatric patients after discharge from community hospitals and then assessed the prevalence of their violent behavior for one year. During that time, 18 percent of the patients who were not abusing alcohol or drugs and 31 percent who were abusing alcohol or drugs committed violent acts. Although the authors did not include a detailed description of the violence in their original publication, they later published data showing that the 951 individuals had committed 608 separate acts of serious violence, including sexual assault, assault causing physical injury, use of a weapon, and six homicides.[23]

This alarming amount of violent behavior occurred despite the fact that the selection process for the study excluded those with the most potential to be violent, including patients who were in jail, homeless, or otherwise not being treated at the start of the study. It also did not include the 44 percent of patients with schizophrenia who were asked but refused to participate, the 20 percent of all subjects who dropped out during the study, or most patients with anosognosia, since patients had to consent to participate. As one critic politely summarized it, "the representativeness of the MacArthur sample would appear to be skewed."[24]

In addition to assessing the prevalence of violence among the patients, the MacArthur study assessed the prevalence of violence among a random selection of community residents in the same neighborhoods where the patients were living. The authors acknowledged that "many of their neighborhoods were disproportionately impoverished and had higher violent crime rates than the city as a whole." The psychiatric patients committed more violent acts than the community residents, but the difference did not achieve statistical significance. Thus, the authors could claim that the psychiatric patients were not statistically significantly more violent than their neighbors. A more accurate summary of the findings would be as follows: if you select seriously mentally ill patients who are being treated at the time of selection, omitting those who are most likely to be violent, and place them in a low-income, crime-ridden neighborhood, they will commit only a few more violent acts than their neighbors.

The most important finding of the MacArthur violence study received little attention. In the original paper, the authors reported that the prevalence of violence committed by patients in the ten-week period prior to their hospitalization and treatment, as obtained by interviews with them, was approximately twice the average prevalence for five ten-week periods after hospitalization, suggesting that treatment had reduced violent behavior by half. In a subsequent report published three years later, they confirmed that treatment had had a major effect in reducing violence. Among patients who attended seven or more treatment sessions in a ten-week period (and who, therefore, were presumably taking medication), only 3 percent became violent during the following ten-week period. Among those who did not attend any treatment sessions, 14 percent became violent in the following ten-week period, a more than fourfold increase.[25] This is one of the clearest demonstrations to date that treating severely mentally ill individuals leads to a dramatic decrease in violence.

Other mental health professionals have used a variety of rationalizations to try to minimize the association of violent behavior and mental illness. Susan Stefan, a lawyer, and her colleagues placed some of the blame for such violence on the individual's relationship with his or her family and social network:

> . . . *violence by persons with a psychiatric diagnosis is grounded in contextual relationships rather than in isolated psychosis. Their lives are set apart by angry or indifferent communities that reject, shun, and sometimes attack them. . . . The contextual nature of violence raises questions of shared culpability. . . .*[26]

In other words, the patients' families and communities are partially to blame for causing the violent behavior.

Other researchers, such as the English psychiatrists Pamela Taylor and John Gunn, have minimized the threat by invoking statistics:

> *On average, every week someone in the UK wins the jackpot on the National Lottery. About 54,999,999 people do not. On average, rather less than one person a week loses their life to a person with mental illness, generally his/her mother, father, sibling, spouse, child or other close contact; 54,999,999 remain safe from this threat.*[27]

One is reminded of Andrew Robertson's 1973 testimony, cited earlier, on the increase in homicides by mentally ill persons in California: "People whom we have released have gone out and killed other people, maimed other people. . . . That sounds bad, but let's qualify it. . . . the odds are still in society's favor."[28]

Resistance to dealing with the problem of violence and mental illness has also been evident at the federal level. As previously noted, a 1977 study in New York State reported that seriously mentally ill individuals had been responsible for 29 percent of homicides in one county during a six-year period. The authors of the study urged that similar studies "should be repeated in other areas to determine whether the apparent increase in violent crime committed by mentally ill perpetrators is indeed a trend."[29] Eight years later, a California study reported that individuals with schizophrenia had committed 10 percent of homicides in one county during a three-year period.[30] Such studies should have been red flags to federal officials, coming as they did in the midst of the emptying of the nation's mental hospitals. Yet not a single additional study of this kind has been undertaken since 1985 by the National Institute of Mental Health or the Center for Mental Health Services, the federal agencies that logically should have done so. To do so, however, would have been politically incorrect. And as public officials well know, you never ask questions to which you do not want the answers.

Other observers have also noted the tendency of mental health professionals to minimize the association of violent behavior and psychiatric illness. One commented that "the profession has become too complacent about the degree of public 'dangerousness' presented by some categories of patient. . . . This complacency has contributed to what yet another enquiry into psychiatric homicide has dubbed 'a scaling down of the perceived level of risk.'" Said another, "No one is served by ignoring the evidence that mental illness is associated with some increased risk for assaultive behavior." Most recently, an Australian psychiatrist trenchantly observed,

> The minimising or dismissal of the correlations between schizophrenia and violence by researchers and academics is less easily explained. In part it is due to misplaced good intentions. Many of us began our research in the area attempting to demonstrate that the public's fear of the violence of people with mental disorders were ill-founded. This they are, in the sense of being exaggerated but not, as it has turned out, in the sense of being groundless. The move to put the increased violence in proper perspective has all too often slid into dismissive minimization.[31]

It is clear that if we ever hope to change psychiatric practices and laws so as to minimize violent behavior by individuals with severe psychiatric disorders, we will first have to educate the professionals themselves.

11 | Fixing the System

The opposition to involuntary committal and treatment betrays a profound misunderstanding of the principle of civil liberties. Medication can free victims from their illness—free them from the Bastille of their psychoses—and restore their dignity, their free will and the meaningful exercise of their liberties.

HERSCHEL HARDIN, 1993

The present treatment system for people with severe psychiatric disorders in the United States is, by any measure, a disaster. The deinstitutionalization movement, implemented half a century ago with the best of intentions and the worst of plans, effectively emptied the nation's public psychiatric hospitals without ensuring that patients would receive care once they left the hospitals.

The disaster is continuing to worsen. In Florida in 1990, there were still 56 state psychiatric beds per 100,000 population; in 2006, this number had been reduced from 56 to 8.[1] In Florida, as in every other state, for those most seriously ill, there are very few beds for treatment as an inpatient and very few resources for treatment as an outpatient.

Clearly, it is time to fix the system. This will require major changes, most of which will not come easily. Civil libertarians will continue to oppose attempts to impose treatment on mentally ill individuals, regardless of how disabled they appear to be, although such opposition is now not as strong as it was in the past. A for-profit system of hospitals and residential settings that has grown skilled at making money by neglecting the most seriously ill patients will also oppose change. And many mental health professionals and administrators simply do not care enough about the problem to work for change. The status quo is always a formidable opponent.

Fixing the system will involve at least the following steps: modification of the laws; identification of the target population; provision and enforcement of treatment; and assessment and research.

Modification of the Laws

The laws governing the treatment of mentally ill individuals were modified beginning in the late 1960s. Through a series of state legislative changes and judicial decisions, the hospitalization and treatment of individuals with severe psychiatric disorders became very difficult to virtually impossible, depending on the state.

Since 1998, the Treatment Advocacy Center (TAC) in Arlington, Virginia, where I am on the board, has led an effort to modify state laws and make them more consistent with what is now known about severe psychiatric disorders. TAC has helped pass assisted outpatient treatment (AOT) laws, which permit the involuntary treatment of seriously mentally ill individuals who are potentially dangerous in the community, in New York (Kendra's Law), California (Laura's Law), and Florida and has helped modify the treatment laws in Maryland, West Virginia, Illinois, Michigan, Minnesota, North Dakota, South Dakota, Montana, Idaho, Wyoming, Utah, Nevada, and Washington. For example, in West Virginia, the criterion for involuntary treatment was broadened so that the person's past history could be considered; in Maryland, the criterion was broadened so that the person no longer had to be "imminently" dangerous.

Despite these successes, much work remains to be done in modifying state laws. Eight states still do not even have a statute allowing AOT: Maine, Massachusetts, Connecticut, New Jersey, Maryland, Tennessee, Nevada, and New Mexico. Most other states that have effective laws are not utilizing them properly.

Identification of the Target Population

In order to fix the system, we must identify the target population. Anecdotally, most people involved in community psychiatric services, jails, and homeless shelters can identify that small group of seriously mentally ill individuals who cause the most problems and regularly rotate among these facilities. They are the "regulars" among hospital readmissions, the "frequent flyers" in the jail system, and the "trouble makers" in the homeless shelters. Many of them are well known to local police, who are often on a first-name basis with them.

Surprisingly little research has been done to precisely quantify this group. In Virginia, 14 percent of psychiatric hospital admissions were said to account for 40 percent of the total hospital costs. In North Carolina, among 1,906 individuals with schizophrenia, "about 20 percent" were reported to be disproportionately responsible for psychiatric hospitalizations, use of emergency psychiatric services, arrests, violence, and victimization. In Massachusetts, among 13,816 individuals receiving psychiatric services from the state, 14 percent were responsible for all "serious violence against persons," and less than 2 percent were responsible for 20 percent of arrests.[2] Another useful study was the previously cited one carried out in England, which determined that, among all individuals with schizophrenia, 10 percent were responsible for 80 percent of the total costs.[3]

As was suggested in chapter 1, the number of seriously ill individuals who are homeless or incarcerated could approach 400,000, which is 10 percent of the estimated total of 4 million seriously mentally ill individuals. Until better data become available, it seems reasonable to use 10 percent as the size of the target population on which to focus attempts to fix the system. Within that 10 percent, an estimated 10 percent of those—or 1 percent of all individuals with serious psychiatric disorders—have likely committed homicides or other violent crimes and have therefore clearly demonstrated a propensity for violent behavior.

The best indicators to use in identifying the potentially most problematic individuals with severe psychiatric disorders are found in studies of violent behavior. Seven identifying factors are most frequently cited: past history of violence; substance abuse; anosognosia with medication noncompliance; antisocial personality disorder; paranoid symptoms; neurological impairment; and gender.

1. *Past history of violence.* A person's past history of violence is the most important predicator of future violence among all people, whether mentally ill or not. In addition, the younger people are when they initially become violent, the more likely they are to be violent later.

2. *Substance abuse.* As has been known for centuries, alcohol makes some people more aggressive. Among individuals with severe psychiatric disorders, alcohol abuse is especially pernicious. In a Finnish study, for example, persons with schizophrenia who abused alcohol were seven times more likely to commit violent crimes than those who did not abuse alcohol. Drugs other than alcohol, especially amphetamines, cocaine, and PCP, may also exacerbate violent tendencies. In an Australian study of individuals with schizophrenia, substance abusers, compared to non–substance abusers, were seven times more likely to be convicted of violent offenses and four times more likely to be convicted of homicides.[4]

3. *Anosognosia with medication noncompliance.* As was discussed in chapter 7, many individuals who are not aware of their illness refuse medication and are liable to become homeless or incarcerated. They are also more apt to become violent, as at least ten separate studies show. For example, in a study of male inpatients with psychosis, "participants who did not generally take their medication engaged in significantly more severe violence." A study of 63 inpatients with schizophrenia reported that "patients who later became violent were, on admission, less compliant [with medication] and had less insight into the necessity for treatment." A study of individuals with schizophrenia found that "treatment noncompliance was ubiquitous among violent patients."

Among 133 outpatients with schizophrenia in another study, those who "had problems with medication compliance" were four times more likely to become violent. A three-year study of almost 2,000 outpatients with schizophrenia-related diagnoses reported that those who refused to take medication were twice as likely to be rehospitalized, arrested, or victimized or to become violent.[5]

4. *Antisocial personality disorder.* Severe psychiatric disorders are equal-opportunity diseases that can affect anyone. They may affect people with a kind and generous personality, but they may also affect people with a preexisting antisocial personality disorder. This condition, which in the past was referred to as sociopathy, is defined as "a pervasive pattern of disregard for, and violation of, the rights of others" and is exhibited by lying, impulsivity, criminal acts, and lack of remorse, among other acts. The combination of a severe psychiatric disorder in an individual with these personality characteristics leads, as would be expected, to more frequent incarceration and violent behavior. The psychologist Sheilagh Hodgins, a prominent English researcher, and her colleagues have shown that individuals with schizophrenia who are violent can be divided into those with an antisocial personality disorder, in which case they became violent prior to developing schizophrenia, and those without an antisocial personality disorder, in which case they became violent only after developing schizophrenia.[6]

5. *Paranoid symptoms.* Multiple studies have suggested that seriously mentally ill individuals who believe that people are following them or trying to hurt them (i.e., are paranoid) are more likely to commit acts of violence, especially against individuals they believe are persecuting them. If you truly believe someone is trying to harm you, it may seem logical to try to harm the other person first. Some researchers have also suggested that a belief that outside forces are controlling your mind, which clinicians refer to as control override, is associated with increased violent behavior. Similarly, claims have been made that command hallucinations—voices that tell you what to do—increase violent behavior, but other studies have not been able to replicate these findings.[7]

6. *Neurological impairment.* Violent behavior is associated with both specific neurological impairment involving brain structures, such as the

amygdala, and brain chemistry, such as the serotonin system. It therefore is not surprising that neurological impairment has been found to be a predictor of violent behavior in individuals with schizophrenia. In one study, inpatients who were persistently violent had more neurological impairment than either those who were transiently violent or those who were not violent. In another study, individuals with schizophrenia who were violent were distinguished by multiple differences in brain function, measured by neuroimaging.[8] For example, in a functional MRI study of violent individuals with schizophrenia compared to nonviolent individuals with schizophrenia, the two groups differed in areas of activation in the frontal and temporal brain areas.

7. *Gender.* Men are responsible for 85–90 percent of violent behavior everywhere in the world; women, for only 10–15 percent. Women with severe psychiatric disorders are the exception to this rule. Two studies of inpatients with psychosis reported that men and women were equally assaultive. Studies of homicides committed by mentally ill individuals have almost uniformly found women to be overrepresented. For example, in Austria women accounted for 31 percent of such homicides, and in New Zealand for 32 percent.[9] Mentally ill women are therefore more likely than would be expected to be included in any list of problematic patients.

Although each of these seven factors may operate independently to help identify mentally ill individuals who are problematic, they also influence each other. Individuals with antisocial personality traits are more likely to abuse drugs, and people who are paranoid are less likely to take medication. The maximum predictive value of these seven factors is achieved when they are used together. In a study of violent acts among seriously mentally ill outpatients in North Carolina, neither substance abuse nor medication noncompliance alone predicted which patients would become violent, but a combination of the two factors did.[10] It seems likely that four of these factors—history of violence; substance abuse; anosognosia with medication noncompliance; and antisocial personality disorder—will identify the vast majority of the most problematic patients when considered together.

Attempts are underway to develop systems to predict which seriously mentally ill individuals are most likely to become violent. Several violence risk assessment scales have been developed and have shown promise, an effort led by the MacArthur Foundation's Violence Risk Assessment Network. John Monahan and Henry Steadman of the MacArthur network have suggested that, by means of predictive factors, mentally ill patients can be classified into four categories of violence risk: low, moderate, high, and very high. It should be remembered, however, that predictors are merely that. As summarized by two researchers in this field, "Like a good weather forecaster, the clinician does not state with certainty that an event will occur . . . [but rather] the likelihood that a future event will occur."[11]

Identifying the target population is useful, of course, only insofar as mental health professionals and police officers are aware of who has been identified. Currently, privacy laws in most states preclude the exchange of critical information. As a result, physicians in emergency rooms often must evaluate psychotic individuals without the benefit of their past history. Similarly, police officers and sheriffs are often called to homes where a seriously mentally ill individual is threatening family members, yet the officer cannot access information regarding the persons' propensity toward violence or other history.

Red-flagging Violent Patients

At the Veterans Administration Medical Center in Portland, Oregon, hospital staff identified forty-eight psychiatric patients who had a history of violent behavior. The hospital computer system red-flagged these individuals so that whenever they appeared for treatment, clinicians and administrative personnel were made aware of their status. Some red flags included specific instructions, such as "hospital police should be asked to stand by until released by examining clinician." During the year prior to the implementation of this system, the forty-eight patients had been responsible for forty-seven violent incidents in the hospital; during the year following its implementation, the number of violent incidents was only four, a 92 percent reduction. The hospital periodically reviews the red-flag status of each patient, and the flag may be removed "if there is clear evidence of cooperative behavior."

D. J. Drummond, L. F. Sparr, and G. H. Gordon, "Hospital violence reduction among high-risk patients," Journal of the American Medical Association 261 (1989): 2531–34.

The solution to this problem is to develop a database listing those individuals with severe psychiatric disorders who have proven dangerous. Names would be added to the list only by judicial order, and it would be restricted to the highest-risk patients. The list undoubtedly would include many of the forty thousand individuals who are the most dangerous. Password-protected, the database would be made available only to authorized mental health professionals, law enforcement officers, and firearms dealers to prevent the sale of guns to at-risk individuals.

In order to be effective, such a list must be available across state lines and would therefore require national legislation. Many severely mentally ill persons migrate from state to state. Officials in each state know some things about them, but nobody knows the person's entire history. An example was Henry Brown, diagnosed with schizophrenia, who was killed in 2004 by officers in California after he shot three people. For twenty years, Brown had migrated across many states, including Mississippi, Georgia, South Carolina, Texas, Ohio, Illinois, and California, in response to voices. He was intermittently hospitalized, jailed, and homeless in most of these states and committed "bizarre crimes that grew increasingly violent" during periods when he was not taking his medication.[12]

Provision and Enforcement of Treatment

Once state laws governing treatment have been modified and the target population identified, it is then necessary to provide treatment and, if needed, enforce it. The treatment of severe mental illnesses involves, first and foremost, the use of antipsychotic medication.

But medication is only part of the treatment plan. An effective system must also include a sufficient number of psychiatric beds for the admission of acutely ill patients and sufficient funding to allow patients to remain long enough to achieve control of their symptoms, normally a period of two to four weeks. Such a system must also include a small number of beds for severely and chronically ill individuals for whom existing medications are not effective. In the past, such beds were provided by state psychiatric hospitals, and some similar provision should be available in every state, both to provide humane care and to function as an asylum, in the best sense of the word, for individuals who are too disabled to protect themselves.

Outpatient psychiatric services must also be readily available. The PACT model, started in Madison, Wisconsin, and described in chapter 6, is both clinically effective and cost-effective and should be implemented nationwide.[13] Outpatient care also includes rehabilitation, vocational training, and housing, all of which can be effectively provided by the much lauded clubhouse model. In clubhouses, mentally ill individuals congregate for socialization and to learn job skills; most clubhouses also contract with businesses to provide jobs for their members and have a housing program. The first clubhouse was Fountain House, which opened in New York City half a century ago and which is still considered to be an excellent program.[14] Like PACT programs, clubhouses should be a common ingredient in psychiatric services nationwide.

But outpatient, rehabilitation, vocation, and housing services are not effective for individuals with severe psychiatric disorders unless such individuals are receiving adequate medication to ameliorate their symptoms. The efficacy of medications to treat severe psychiatric disorders is well established. Medications do not *cure* these disorders, but they can help control the symptoms.

The major types of medications available for use are antipsychotics (such as risperidone), mood stabilizers (such as lithium), and antidepressants (such as fluoxetine). Their effectiveness derives, at least in part, from their ability to affect specific brain chemicals, especially neurotransmitters, which carry information between brain cells. Insofar as a patient's violent behavior is caused by psychotic symptoms such as paranoid delusions, the reduction of those symptoms usually produces a reduction in violent behavior. A two-year study of aggression in individuals with schizophrenia found that "the day-by-day decline of aggressive incidents after the start of neuroleptic [antipsychotic] treatment was highly significant. . . . The results support the assumption that neuroleptics [antipsychotics] are not only effective in controlling violent outbursts . . . but also in preventing violence in schizophrenia." Similarly, a study of adolescents with bipolar disorder reported that those who did not take medication committed criminal acts almost five times more frequently than those who did take medication.[15]

In addition to being effective in controlling psychotic symptoms, some medications have been claimed to specifically reduce aggressive behavior. Evidence is strong to support this claim for clozapine (Clozaril), an antipsychotic used widely in Europe and China but less widely in the United States. Its lower use in this country is related both to the fact that patients' blood must be regularly monitored to prevent side effects and to the fact that in recent years clozapine has been off-patent and thus available generically, thereby decreasing interest in the pharmaceutical industry in pushing its use. But it is effective. In one study, for example, "the patients [with psychosis] who received clozapine had lower rates of arrest than the patients who never received clozapine"; in addition, "the arrests rates of the patients taking clozapine were significantly lower while they were taking the drug than before they were given the drug."[16] Clearly, clozapine should be the antipsychotic of choice for severely mentally ill individuals who exhibit violent behavior.

Claims have been made that other drugs have specific anti-aggressive effects, but evidence to support these claims is much weaker than is the evidence for clozapine. These drugs include other antipsychotics, mood stabilizers, and a class of drugs called beta-blockers. Many studies of the anti-aggression effects of these drugs are of questionable validity because the pharmaceutical companies that made the drugs funded the studies.

Given the role of substance abuse in exacerbating violent behavior in individuals with severe psychiatric disorders, it is important to utilize all possible treatment methods to minimize such abuse. Disulfiram (Antabuse), which leads to unpleasant side effects when alcohol is ingested; naltrexone (Revia, Vivitrol); and methadone, which blocks the effects of heroin, are moderately effective and should be used. In addition, given the importance of anosognosia as a cause of not taking medication, it would be extremely useful if there were effective treatments for this problem. Approximately one-third of individuals with anosognosia regain some insight into their illness in the course of being treated with antipsychotic or mood-stabilizing drugs, but the other two-thirds do not. Efforts to improve insight in such individuals have failed, including the use of videotapes to show recovering patients what they looked like when they were acutely psychotic.[17]

Although effective medications are available, they work only if people take them. Malcolm Tate, Herb Mullin, Bryan Stanley, and other seriously mentally ill persons who have little or no insight into their illness see no need to take medication. In such cases, involuntary treatment is the only solution.

Involuntarily treating individuals with severe psychiatric disorders is adamantly opposed by some civil libertarians, lawyers, and mental health professionals, who argue that coercion is rarely, if ever, justified. By contrast, members of the general public recognize the need for such involuntarily treatment. A national survey reported that 87 percent of public respondents "said that mentally ill homeless should be sent to mental hospitals even when they don't want to go." Another national survey found the public willing to involuntarily commit a person with schizophrenia to a hospital if that person was a danger to self (91 percent said yes) or a danger to others (95 percent said yes).[18]

Uncivil Liberties

The remedy is treatment—most essentially, medication. In most cases, this means involuntary treatment because people in the throes of their illness have little or no insight into their own condition. If you think you are Jesus Christ or an avenging angel, you are not likely to agree that you need to go to the hospital.

Anti-treatment advocates insist that involuntary committal should be limited to cases of imminent physical danger—instances where a person is going to do serious bodily harm to himself or to somebody else. But the establishment of such "dangerousness" usually comes too late—a psychotic break or loss of control, leading to violence, happens suddenly. And all the while, the victim suffers the ravages of the illness itself, the degradation of life, the tragic loss of individual potential.

The anti-treatment advocates say: "If that's how people want to live (babbling on a street corner, in rags), or if they wish to take their own lives, they should be allowed to exercise their free will. To interfere—with involuntary committal—is to deny them their civil liberties." As for the tragedy that follows from this dictum, well, "That's the price that has to be paid if society is to maintain its civil liberties."

Whether or not anti-treatment advocates actually voice such opinions, they seem content to sacrifice a few lives here and there to uphold an abstract doctrine. Their intent, if noble, has a chilly, Stalinist justification—the odd tragedy along the way is warranted to ensure the greater good.

Herschel Hardin, op-ed, **Vancouver Sun, July 22, 1993.**

There are many methods for ensuring that people with severe psychiatric disorders take medications, and almost all of them are effective. Informal methods include using a person's disability payments as leverage. The vast majority of individuals with severe psychiatric disorders receive monthly disability benefits through Social Security or the Veterans Administration. For those who are disabled, the court can appoint a "representative payee," who can insist that the person follow a specific treatment plan, including taking medication, as a condition for receiving part of the money. Studies have shown that the use of representative payees decreases alcohol and drug abuse and markedly decreases psychiatric readmissions to hospitals.[19]

A second method of informal leverage involves making access to good housing conditional on following a treatment plan. Housing for mentally ill individuals living on disability payments is grossly inadequate throughout the United States, so being able to access the limited supply of special housing is a strong incentive. A survey of five cities found that housing had been used as leverage for approximately one-third of mentally ill persons.[20] Until an adequate supply of housing is available, this method of leverage is likely to be used.

A third method of informal leverage is used for mentally ill individuals charged with crimes, usually misdemeanors. Individuals who meet the criteria are assigned to specialized courts known as mental health courts. These courts are now available in at least thirty-four states, and one study found that 92 percent of them "reported using jail as a sanction for noncompliance" with treatment. The judge, in effect, says, You can either comply with your treatment plan, or you can go to jail—your choice. As would be expected, this method of enforcing treatment is effective. A study of a mental health court in Washington State reported that, among participants, arrests decreased from 119 to 34, and arrests for assault or other violent crimes decreased from 12 to 2, over a six-month period. A study of a mental health court in Pittsburgh reported that it not only reduced jail time but also saved taxpayers $3.5 million over a two-year period.[21]

There are also formal mechanisms for compelling treatment. One method makes use of conservatorships, under which a court appoints a person to make decisions for a legally incompetent individual. These are often used for individuals with mental retardation or dementia but have not been widely used for individuals with mental illness.

Conditional release, under which persons who have been committed to psychiatric hospitals can be released on the condition that they continue taking medication and otherwise follow their treatment plan, is much more common. If they do not comply, they can be involuntarily hospitalized. A study in New Hampshire, where conditional release has been widely used, found that the program led to markedly increased medication compliance, decreased rehospitalization, and decreased substance abuse, as well as a reduction in violent episodes by half.[22]

A variant form of conditional release widely used in Oregon is the Psychiatric Security Review Board (PSRB), which has legal jurisdiction over mentally ill individuals charged with crimes. The PSRB has been rightfully praised as a cost-effective way to reduce violence and other criminal behavior. In one study, mentally ill individuals were reported to have only one-quarter as many contacts with the police when under the jurisdiction of the PSRB compared with when they were not under the board's jurisdiction.[23]

The most widely publicized method of compelling treatment is the use of assisted outpatient treatment (AOT). In other countries, AOT is referred to as a community treatment order. Like conditional release, AOT allows mentally ill persons to live in the community only if they follow their treatment plan, including taking their medications. If they do not, in most states the person can be involuntarily hospitalized. The main difference between conditional release and AOT is that the former must follow a hospitalization, whereas the latter can be initiated for an individual currently living in the community. The criteria for implementing AOT vary by state; forty-two states have some AOT provision, but only a minority use it. At the Treatment Advocacy Center we have developed a model AOT law; it is available on our website, www.treatmentadvocacycenter.org.

Assessments of AOT have found it to be remarkably effective. The most detailed studies were conducted in North Carolina and New York. In the latter, a provision for AOT was implemented in 1999 and called Kendra's Law after Kendra Webdale, who was killed by a man with untreated schizophrenia.[24]

The effect of AOT on medication compliance has been to double it. In New York, for example, 34 percent of patients regularly took medication prior to AOT, but 69 percent did so after being placed on AOT. This level of compliance produced a marked decrease in psychiatric hospital readmissions and total hospital days. AOT's reduction of psychiatric admissions and hospital days is evident in the six studies summarized in table 1. Another well-designed study, in North Carolina, carried out by Drs. Marvin Swartz and Jeffrey Swanson at Duke

Table 1.

Effects of Assisted Outpatient Treatment (AOT) on Psychiatric Admissions

	Number of psychiatric admissions per year		Number of hospital days per year	
	Before AOT	On AOT	Before AOT	On AOT
New York[24]	3.1	N/A	100	44
District of Columbia[25]	1.8	1.0	55	38
North Carolina[26]	1.4	0.3	22	14
Ohio[27]	1.5	0.4	133	44
Iowa[28]	1.3	0.3	33	5
North Carolina[29]	1.2	0.3	33	5

University and their colleagues, randomized patients with psychosis to either AOT or services as usual; those maintained on AOT for more than six months had fewer hospital admissions (0.3 vs. 1.2) and fewer hospital days (5 vs. 33) per year.[24–29]

AOT has also been shown to decrease other adverse effects of deinstitutionalization. In New York, AOT reduced homelessness among severely mentally ill persons from 19 percent to 5 percent.[30] In North Carolina, AOT decreased the chances of being victimized, from 42 percent to 24 percent. The researchers speculated on possible reasons for this:

> By facilitating adherence and ensuring more consistent follow-up, outpatient commitment may lead to reduced symptoms, better functioning in social relationships, and improved judgment. In turn, these changes should lessen a person's vulnerability to abuse by others and lower the probability of becoming involved in dangerous situations where victimization is more likely.[31]

Two studies have also assessed the effect of AOT on arrest rates. In North Carolina, a randomized study reported that patients "with a prior history of multiple hospitalizations combined with prior arrests and/or violent behavior" had a reduction in arrests from 45 percent to 12 percent in one year while participating in AOT.[32] In New York, the percentage of mentally ill individuals arrested decreased from 30 percent to 5 percent, and the percentage of those incarcerated decreased from 23 percent to 3 percent while on AOT.[33] In both studies, AOT was also accompanied by a major reduction in alcohol and drug abuse.

Finally, two studies have assessed the effect of AOT on violent behavior. In a randomized trial in North Carolina, subjects with a history of serious violence had a reduction in violence from 42 percent to 27 percent when the AOT was continued for at least six months.[34] In New York, AOT reduced the proportion of individuals who "physically harmed others" from 15 percent to 8 percent, and the proportion who "threatened physical harm" from 28 percent to 16 percent.[35]

The consistency of findings regarding the effectiveness of AOT is impressive. Only one U.S. study, in fact, did not find significant effects. In that study, there were no consequences for patients who did not take their medication, so it would seem it was not a true test of AOT.[36]

Despite its success, AOT is still not widely used. In New York State, for example, AOT was implemented on only 6,013 individuals between its inception in 1999 and mid-2007.[37] Resistance to using all forms of involuntary treatment remains high among mental health professionals. In addition, opponents of involuntary treatment have written extensively about its purported adverse effects on individuals forced to undergo it. Multiple studies, however, have shown that the majority of patients forced to take medication will, in retrospect, acknowledge that it was necessary. In one study, for example, seventeen of twenty-four involuntarily medicated patients "felt that their treatment refusal had been correctly overridden by staff and that they should be treated against their will again if necessary."[38] In the analysis of AOT under Kendra's Law in New York, "62 percent of AOT recipients reported that, all things considered, being court-ordered into treatment has been a good thing for them."[39]

Violence Comes to NAMI

On June 29, 1986, Don Richardson was in Washington, D.C., being installed as president of the National Alliance for the Mentally Ill, now called NAMI. At home in Los Angeles, his son Bill had just finished dinner with his mother. Bill, diagnosed with schizophrenia, had had twenty-six psychiatric admissions in the preceding seven years and had stopped taking his medication six weeks before. Bill heard command hallucinations telling him to kill his mother, so he walked behind her and hit her with a hammer, fracturing her skull in three places. She was not expected to live, but did.

Don Richardson then attempted to get NAMI to speak out on the problem of violence. "To say the mentally ill are no more dangerous than the general population is a statement all of us family members have been parroting for years because we try hard to break the stigma. . . . In our intensity to reduce stigma NAMI is also losing a lot of credibility. . . . Out of the mentally ill population there is no question that there is a segment that is much more violent and to deny that is just reducing the credibility of our movement. . . . I believe it is time for NAMI members to come all the way out of the closet."

Don Richardson, "On violence and forgiveness: A father confronts his fears," NAMI Advocate, May/June 1992; Rael Jean Isaac and Virginia Armat, Madness in the Streets: How Psychiatry and the Law Abandoned the Mentally Ill (New York: Free Press, 1990), pp. 270–78.

So we know how to identify individuals with severe psychiatric disorders who are most in need of treatment, including those who are most dangerous to themselves and others. We have effective medications to treat them, and we have mechanisms, both formal and informal, to compel treatment. One major problem remains: How can we be sure these people actually take their medication?

One simple, but labor-intensive, means for ensuring treatment compliance is to observe the person taking the medication. This is widely used for patients with tuberculosis who are unable to, or refuse to, take their anti-tuberculous medication regularly. Inconsistent medication encourages the emergence of treatment-resistant strains of the tuberculous bacteria as well as the exposure of the public to persons who may spread the disease. This has led to the widespread use of directly observed therapy (DOT), which has been shown to be cost-effective. Patients with tuberculosis who still refuse to take medication under DOT can be involuntarily hospitalized and treated for several months until they are no longer infectious.[40]

A less expensive but highly effective means of ensuring medication compliance is to give the medication by long-acting injection. Three antipsychotics with a long-acting form are available in the United States, and others are available in Europe. They need to be given by injection every three or four weeks. Attempts are also underway to develop a small medication capsule that can be placed beneath the skin, where it will slowly release antipsychotic medication over several months.

Finally, means are available, and can be further developed, to measure medications in a person's blood or urine to ensure they are being taken. Many mood stabilizers and antipsychotics can already be measured. For those that cannot, it is possible to add to the pills a substance such as riboflavin, which is then detectable in the person's urine.[41] Similar measures have been used to monitor medication compliance for tuberculosis and could be instituted to monitor the treatment of severe psychiatric disorders.

Guaranteed Medication?

On July 12, 1976, Edward Allaway, a janitor at Cal State Fullerton, walked into the university library with a rifle and opened fire, killing seven people and injuring two others. Allaway, suffering from paranoid schizophrenia, feared that people were trying to put a bomb in his car and kill him. Five years earlier, he had been hospitalized for delusions. Allaway was found not guilty by reason of insanity and hospitalized.

Since 1999, his attorney has claimed that he has been in full remission while not on medication and should therefore be released. Many have opposed his release under any circumstances. Others have argued that patients like Allaway should be released only on medication and under circumstances in which it is guaranteed that he will always have to take his medication.

S. Pfeifer, "Mass killer says he's no longer mentally ill," Los Angeles Times, June 5, 2001

Assessment and Research

The final ingredient in fixing the system is assessment and research. Mental health programs at the local and the state levels should collect regular data on the number of seriously mentally ill individuals who are homeless, jailed, victimized, and violent. These data should then be used to assess the effectiveness of their treatment programs. The federal government could require data as a condition for the annual federal grants given to each state or for eligibility for Medicaid reimbursement. The data could also be used to hold public mental health officials responsible when programs fail.

The federal government should play an important role in research on these issues. More research is needed to determine the best methods for identifying the target population; improved methods for assessing anosognosia; predictors of violent behavior; better pharmacological treatments for reducing violent behavior; and the relative effectiveness of assisted outpatient treatment (AOT) versus other methods of leveraging treatment. Funding for these types of research has been virtually nonexistent among federal agencies. A rare exception occurred in early 2007, when the National Institute of Mental Health announced a $2 million award to the Nathan Kline Institute for Psychiatric Research to study brain changes in individuals with schizophrenia who become violent. This is an excellent example of the kind of research the federal government should be supporting.

Ultimately, the question is not whether we have the means to identify and treat the subgroup of mentally ill individuals who are most problematic. We clearly do. The question, rather, is whether we have the will to do so. And if we do not have the will now, how much worse must the disaster become before we acquire the will?

12 | Coda: Death by the Roadside

*Our present policy of discharging helpless human beings to a
hostile community is immoral and inhumane. It is a return to
the Middle Ages, when the mentally ill roamed the streets and
little boys threw rocks at them.*

ROBERT REICH, 1973

C hester, South Carolina, is not the best town for black people to go
on trial. The county courthouse, built in 1832, has two imposing,
twenty-two-step staircases ascending to a hexacolumn portico that frames
the courthouse entrance. A Confederate cannon stands on the lawn beneath
massive old trees. Nearby is a Confederate memorial to those who fought:
"Their fame increases like the branches of a tree through the hidden course
of time." General William Tecumseh Sherman burned almost everything
in sight when he passed through Chester in the spring of 1865, to the
delight of the area slaves, including Lothell Tate's great-grandfather.

On May 24, 1989, a late spring day with temperatures in the eight-
ies, Lothell Tate went on trial for the murder of Malcom Tate, her
brother. Although the family had lived in North Carolina, the homicide had occurred in South Carolina. A farmer driving a tractor had
spotted Tate's body three days after the killing. A receipt found at the
scene led to Malcom's identification, and two days later Pauline Wilk-

197

erson and Lothell Tate were charged with his murder. It was the day
before Christmas Eve.

According to the newspaper, Lothell wore "a crisp white dress with
lace-trimmed collar and cuffs" for the trial. Her mother, scheduled to
go on trial later, "sat behind her daughter and listened quietly, dabbing
her eyes with a tissue." Lothell's daughter, N'Zinga, and three of Lothell's
brothers attended part of the proceedings. The jury consisted of five
men and seven women, equally divided between blacks and whites.
News of the trial competed with the arrival of Mike Wallace, in town
to do a show for *Sixty Minutes* investigating why the son of a prominent Chester family had been merely fined and put under house arrest
after being convicted of cocaine distribution and bookmaking.

Lothell took the stand and explained why she had killed her
brother:

> *I was just saying to myself this is the only thing I know to do, that we done
> asked people to help us and we done begged people to help us and nobody
> did anything and I was scared that one day Malcoum was going to lose his
> mind and harm me and my daughter and I just didn't know what else to
> do because it had been years we had been asking for help; it ain't been like
> we just started asking for help the last six months; it had been years. Mal-
> coum had been sick since he was nineteen years old and he was thirty some-
> thing and every time we asked somebody to help us, they said we can't do
> anything until he gets violent and I just couldn't imagine him hurting my
> daughter or me or even my mother and then what would happen to him if
> he killed somebody else or hurt somebody else.*[1]

Lothell attempted to describe the stress and terror of living, month after
month, year after year, with someone who she believed was going to
kill her daughter, but the task of explaining this was a daunting one.

The prosecutor, eponymously named John R. Justice, made short
work of Lothell's testimony. Highly experienced, Justice was regarded
as one of the best prosecutors in the state and was later elected president
of the National District Attorneys Association. He emphasized to the
jury that a crime committed in self-defense or in defense of another

person could be justified only "under the immediate and imminent danger of losing their own life or suffering grave bodily injury." In other words, it was not enough that Malcoum had threatened to kill them and stood over them in the middle of the night; he must also have been poised with knife in hand to justify Lothell's act.

Lothell had made a statement to the police confessing to the crime. The statement was read in court, causing her to sob openly. According to a newspaper account, "Mrs. Wilkerson wept quietly," and N'Zinga, Lothell's eight-year-old daughter, "stuck her fingers in her ears." One of Lothell's brothers told the reporter later that "she just didn't want to hear that."[2]

The prosecutor elicited sympathy for Malcoum. He referred to him as having "trusting innocence" toward his family but who "was scorned by much of his family." Malcoum was said to be "not violent" and "offered society no harm." Lothell, by contrast, was in Justice's estimation "something worse than a vicious person, she is a sanctimonious person who sets herself up to decide the issue of life and death of another human being and that's worse than viciousness." Justice called Malcoum's killing an "execution" for merely "kicking in the front door of his mother's house when they wouldn't let him in." In closing, Justice compared Lothell's actions to those of the German Nazis: "That form of thinking, Ladies and Gentlemen, is called fascism where we do away [with] and extinguish groups of people because we don't like something about them or because they annoy us or we don't like living with them." He told the jury that he was not seeking the death penalty, because the "circumstances of aggravation set out in the law" were not present. But he concluded, "There is only one verdict in this case, guilty of murder. Please do your duty."

Lothell Tate's court-appointed lawyer, Tyre Lee, presented a stark contrast to the prosecutor. Proud of his South Carolina heritage, Lee had graduated from the University of South Carolina School of Law thirteen years before. He was in private practice in Chester, and his work as a public defender paid considerably less than his private work. Years later, when Lee ran for the prosecutor's position, he was soundly defeated by his opponent, with 73 percent of the vote to 27 percent.

Lee exhibited little interest in Lothell Tate's case. According to her testimony in a later appeal, "I called Mr. Lee in January, February, and March. I never got him. I got his secretary or his answering service, and I left messages. He never called me back." Finally, in the month prior to the scheduled trial, Lee saw Lothell twice for "maybe about 45 minutes to an hour" each time.

Tyre Lee's defense of Lothell Tate was *de minimis*. In addition to putting Lothell on the stand, he called three of her brothers as witnesses. Each of them verified her story and described Malcoum's repeated threats to kill her daughter.

Lee made no attempt to present other available evidence regarding Malcoum's proven dangerousness. The records of Malcoum's two hospitalizations in Maryland and three hospitalizations in North Carolina clearly described him as a danger to himself and others. They included notations of his violent tirade in the hospital emergency room, his threats to kill his mother and other members of the family, and comments such as "God had told him to kill everybody." But Lee apparently did not request those records.

One person Lee could have called to testify was Eugene Maloney, the psychiatric director of the mental health center in Gastonia, where Malcoum had been intermittently treated as an outpatient. Well trained and experienced, Maloney had testified in over one hundred murder trials. A month before the trial, Maloney was quoted in a newspaper article sympathizing with the defendant: "There's just so much you can do if you've got an out-of-control, hallucinating, paranoid-schizophrenic in the house." Maloney added that patients like Malcoum were being discharged from the state hospital before being stabilized and that "by having these patients sent back in the community, it puts the whole community at risk." Since Maloney knew Malcoum's case personally, he was potentially an important witness. Maloney called Tyre Lee's office prior to the trial and was willing to testify, but Lee did not return the call.[3]

Lothell Tate asked Mr. Lee to call three other witnesses in her defense, but he declined to do so. One was Harvey Morton, the manager of the fitness center where Malcoum Tate regularly worked out.

Three months prior to the trial, in a newspaper article, Morton had described Malcoum as dangerous; he said he never sat with his back to Malcoum "because you never knew when Malcoum would blow." Another potential witness was John Baggett, executive director of the North Carolina Alliance for the Mentally Ill. Baggett also had a severely mentally ill son and offered to testify. I was the third witness Lothell Tate asked to have called. I had written to her on March 2, 1989, offering to testify without charge in her defense. Lothell replied that she had given my name to Tyre Lee, adding, "He said he'd call you and talk with you about coming to the trial." He never did. Lee later claimed that he didn't call any of these witnesses, because "their testimony would not be relevant in this particular case."[4]

In fact, there was much potential testimony that was highly relevant to the case. The jury could have been told about cases like Vincent Gillette's, who in 1984 at age eighteen had killed his older brother Steven in Philadelphia. Steven, severely mentally ill, had broken his brother's arm twice, chased his mother with a knife, wrecked the furniture, and attempted to set the house on fire. Steven's family was terrified of him, but "his family had been turned away, again and again, by hospitals, schools, police, and the mental health system itself in its attempts to get treatment for the young man." Desperate, Ms. Gillette had "warned mental health professionals that she would kill Steven if she had to." Vincent did it for her. When he was sentenced for manslaughter to a minimum sentence of five years, the judge said, "You had a lot of justification for what you did. . . . You did everything in your power to get help, but society didn't give you any."[5]

The jury also could have learned about LaVoy Gliddon, a pharmacist in Genoa, Illinois, who in 1986 had killed his son. The son, diagnosed with paranoid schizophrenia, was extremely violent and had attacked his parents on numerous occasions, causing brain damage and epilepsy in his mother after he hit her with the butt of a rifle. He had been psychiatrically hospitalized and jailed on numerous occasions, but the authorities would not keep him in treatment. The family, according to Mrs. Gliddon, had "lived in fear of our lives for the past eleven years, hooked up directly to the Genoa Police Station with alarm buttons to push on each of the three levels of our home in the event that our son would attack us."[6]

In addition to cases similar to the Tate case, the jury could have been told what it was like to live with a severely mentally ill but untreated family member. In 1984, for example, Jim and Maggie Phillips had been held hostage in their own home by their son, who had bipolar disorder:

> *There, he tyrannized his parents with hostile and bizarre behavior, they said. He exploded in anger if his father watched TV or his mother sang. He knocked sconces and shelves from the walls and smashed glassware.*
>
> *His father retreated more and more to his room; his mother sought peace in church or nearby parks.*
>
> *"The more I backed off, the more I feared him," she recalled. "If he would get up and go out, I would run downstairs and try to fix my husband something to eat real fast. I could hardly get anything done before he would get back in the door and I'd get caught. . . . He had me terrified."*

The Phillipses repeatedly "asked for help from city mental health and law enforcement officials" but received none. Eventually, they simply moved out, leaving their home to their son. He then "set fires on the lawn, erected obscene posters, discarded the light fixtures and most of the doors, bashed in the gas range and stripped every inch of wallpaper in the house."[7]

Unfortunately, the jury did not have an opportunity to hear these or similar stories that might have helped them understand what Lothell Tate and her family had gone through. Tyre Lee, in fact, did not even present a closing statement at the trial.

The jury deliberated for about an hour and, as expected, found Lothell Tate guilty of murder. Judge Don Rushing, a former state senator, added for the record that, although he was the judge and thus "not permitted to have an opinion about the facts in a case," he did have an opinion. Lothell's crime, he said, "was as brutal and as dispassionate a murder as I have had the opportunity to see as a trial judge." He sentenced Lothell to life in prison, for which she would have to serve a minimum of twenty years. She was immediately taken into custody. Pauline Wilkerson was observed "crying afterward" and was "the only family member in the courtroom when the two-day trial ended."[8]

Pauline Wilkerson's own trial, which took place two months later, was a postscript. The State of South Carolina was apparently reluctant to put a poor, sixty-two-year-old woman in prison for life. In a plea deal arranged by a defense lawyer different from Lothell's, charges against Pauline were reduced to accessory to the murder and withholding evidence. Judge Rushing sentenced her to ten years in prison but reduced it to one year plus five years' probation. She served six months in minimum security in the same prison as her daughter. "They treated me good down there," she told me. "They kept asking me, what are you doing here?"[9]

Lothell Tate appealed her sentence, first at the local level and eventually to the South Carolina Supreme Court. She claimed that her counsel had been inadequate and that her lawyer had failed to call witnesses who could have helped her case. In her appeal, she wrote, "I feel and felt then my brother should have been in the hospital where he could have been watched and taken care of properly. The police and hospital said they couldn't do anything until he hurt someone. I just couldn't let that happen to my daughter or family."

On November 19, 1990, Lothell Tate's first appeal was dismissed. On August 1, 1991, her second appeal was dismissed. On April 14, 1992, her final appeal was dismissed by the state supreme court. With all hope gone for getting out of prison before serving the minimum sentence of twenty years, Lothell Tate stopped her treatment for diabetes. The complications of her illness became increasingly severe, and she died in the South Carolina State Prison on March 28, 1994.

I first met Pauline Wilkerson on October 6, 2004. She was a young-looking seventy-two years old, living in Gastonia with her son Garnell in a modest house next to a factory. A Bible lay on the living room table next to pictures of her children. Young Lothell looked out, smiling, missing a front tooth, with large glasses. Mrs. Wilkerson was continuing to work as a domestic, as she had most of her life. She had applied to live at the Senior Citizen Center but had been rejected because of her felony conviction. Most of her family and friends had stood behind her, she said, because they knew what she had gone through.

North Carolina Today

In the years since Pauline Wilkerson and her daughter killed Malcoum Tate, services for people with severe psychiatric disorders have gotten worse in North Carolina, as they have in most other states. Although assisted outpatient treatment (AOT) is used on a small number of patients in a few counties, its use has not become sufficiently widespread to make much of a difference. In 2000, a report described the state's $2.3 billion psychiatric treatment system as being in total collapse. In 2001, the state legislature instituted a major overhaul, shifting much of the responsibility and funds to private agencies, but by 2005 an analysis concluded that "there is little proof that treatment has improved, and there is growing evidence that the state's complex system of care is worse than ever."[10]

Psychiatric beds to stabilize severely ill patients have decreased in number each year. For those that still exist, there is tremendous pressure on hospital workers to discharge patients prematurely to make room for other patients on the waiting list. Many of the discharged patients then relapse and need rehospitalization, perpetuating the cycle. A 2007 survey reported that almost 12 percent of individuals discharged from the state hospitals were readmitted within a month. It cited a woman in her forties who had been admitted more than one hundred times. Another woman, admitted for suicidal intent and labeled as "clearly a danger to herself," was discharged two days later and promptly committed suicide.[11]

In desperation, North Carolina has given up even trying to stabilize discharged patients in community housing and started dropping them off at homeless shelters. In 2000, the state discharged 763 patients to shelters; by 2004, the number had risen to 1,140. The Rescue Mission in Durham now has an employee specifically assigned to dispense medication to the mission's mentally ill residents.[12] The results of this purging of mentally ill individuals from the psychiatric hospitals into homeless shelters is visible on the streets of Charlotte, Durham, Raleigh, Winston-Salem, and other cities and towns.

The county jails in North Carolina have also become filled with mentally ill persons. In 2006, among the Henderson County Jail's 151 inmates, "head nurse Karen Styles estimated that 90 had some degree of mental illness . . . [of which] 24 have major mental health medications that they are on." "I call it little Broughton [State Hospital] without the medications," she said. Styles described the problems caused by the mentally ill inmates. One with a history of severe violence "was constantly threatening to kill the officers and other inmates." Another, calling himself "the archangel," claimed he could take his eyeballs out and was threatening suicide.[13]

The large number of untreated mentally ill individuals in the community also strains the resources of local police and sheriffs. In the town of Asheboro, which normally has five patrol officers during the day, the police in 2006 were averaging twenty psychiatric involuntary commitment procedures per month. Each commitment averaged three to five hours, but, according to the Asheboro police chief, "it's not unusual for calls to take 11 or 12 hours, and one recent commitment took 21 hours. . . . What that does is take an officer off of the streets and takes them away from being able to answer [other] calls." In Forsyth County, sheriff's deputies may be required to drive as many as eight patients a day to the state hospital, a two-hour trip.[14]

The most tragic effect of increasing number of individuals with severe, untreated psychiatric disorders is homicides. Some of these involved law enforcement officers:

- **1995, Winston-Salem:** George Page, diagnosed with bipolar disorder, fatally shot the police officer Steven Amos as Amos got out of his police car. Amos was coming to Page's apartment house to investigate a report of shots being fired.

- **1999, Hanover County:** John York, diagnosed with schizophrenia but not taking his medication, was shot and killed by police when he advanced toward them with two large knives. The police were attempting to serve commitment papers.

The victims were often selected at random, and sometimes multiple victims were involved:

- **1995, Chapel Hill:** Wendell Williamson, a University of North Carolina law student who was diagnosed with paranoid schizophrenia but not taking medication, shot to death two people picked at random in downtown Chapel Hill.
- **2003, Gastonia:** Keith Hall, diagnosed with paranoid schizophrenia, and with a history of multiple hospitalizations, killed four people during a robbery. Although only twenty-four years old, Hall's police record was thirty-two pages long.

Other homicides were caused by the inappropriate placement of violent mentally ill patients in community facilities:

- **2003, Greensboro:** Carl Porter, who had previously been psychiatrically hospitalized for threatening President Clinton, killed Russell Lane, who had hemiplegia, by stabbing him forty-eight times. Both men were residents of an assisted living facility.
- **2005, Alamance County:** Anthony Zichi, a twenty-five-year-old man with severe mental illness, stabbed to death an eighty-eight-year-old woman who lived in the same group home. Even though Zichi had two previous convictions for assault, he "had been placed by authorities in the small family-care home for the elderly."[15]

As always, however, the most frequent victims were family members of the mentally ill persons.

- **2001, Wilmington:** Matthew Coleman, diagnosed with schizophrenia, bludgeoned his mother to death with a baseball bat.

- **2004, Fayetteville:** David Graham, diagnosed with paranoid schizophrenia, stabbed his father to death.
- **2006, Mecklenburg:** David Crespi, a senior vice president at Wachovia who was being inadequately treated for bipolar disorder, stabbed to death his five-year-old twin daughters while he was "in the midst of a psychotic episode."
- **2007, Clayton:** John Violette, diagnosed with paranoid schizophrenia but not taking his medication, stabbed to death and decapitated his four-year-old daughter.[16]

Tragedies like these are no longer unusual in North Carolina or in any other state. The majority of states, in fact, have worse psychiatric services than North Carolina. In all states, a small minority of individuals with severe psychiatric disorders live in the community untreated and terrify and terrorize others, especially their families. Mental health officials say that nothing can be done unless . . . until . . . their rights . . . the law . . . the words linger in the air, harbingers of a coming storm.

Most families suffer silently. Every few months, however, somewhere in the United States, people like Pauline Wilkerson and Lothell Tate decide to act. Faced with what appears to be inevitable, the unthinkable become thinkable.

- **Virginia, 2003:** Lester Richardson shot to death his son, diagnosed with schizophrenia. The son was described as "evil personified," had terrorized his family, and was also a sexual predator. He had been institutionalized for several years, but mental health officials said they could do nothing more. After the shooting, the court was given letters from forty people, testifying "to what Richardson and his late wife had been through." The judge, in pronouncing a sentence of eight years, said, "I cannot imagine the situation you were in."[17]

Others retrospectively wish they had acted.

- **Nevada, 2004:** Richard Lentino strangled his mother, then stabbed to death his sister and her one-year-old son. Lentino had been "in the top of his high school class" until he developed bipolar disorder. He had recently stopped taking his medication. Lentino's father, a lawyer, when told of the slayings, said, "If I had [had] any clue this would happen, I would have gone over there, killed my son, and turned myself in. . . . It's too much for anyone to bear."[18]

Such cases are an extraordinary commentary, perhaps the ultimate commentary, on our failed mental health system. Ronald Tate, Malcoum and Lothell's brother, said it most clearly:

> *There's a whole lot of people out there who are not getting any help. Don't just leave them on their own. Everybody's got a right to live and be happy. The family of mental patients have a right to live, too.*[19]

APPENDIX A:

U.S. Studies of the Prevalence of Serious Violence by Psychiatric Patients Living in the Community

TRIANGLE MENTAL HEALTH SURVEY (NORTH CAROLINA) (Estroff et al., 1994; Estroff and Zimmer, 1993; Swanson et al., 1997)[1]	
Sample and Methods	**Additional Information**
• 169 individuals being discharged from community and state psychiatric hospitals • all had "major psychiatric disorders" • serious violence = assault, threat or use of weapon, sexual assault, murder • violence ascertained by self-report and interview with "significant other"	• 18-month prevalence of serious violence: 14% • an additional 21% threatened but did not commit a violent act • majority of targets were relatives, especially mothers • "individuals with no treatment contact in the past 6 months had significantly higher odds of violence"
WASHINGTON HEIGHTS STUDY (NEW YORK CITY) (Link et al., 1992; Link and Stueve, 1994)[2]	
Sample and Methods	**Additional Information**
• community samples of 367 psychiatric patients and 386 community residents • 30% schizophrenia and other psychoses, 34% major depression, 36% other diagnoses • violence ascertained by self-report	• lifetime prevalence of "hurting someone badly": 　—first contact patients: 19% 　—repeat contact patients: 12% 　—former patients: 17% • lifetime prevalence in random sample of community residents: 5%

	• weapon use in past 5 years also significantly increased in repeat contact and former patients • ". . . only patients with current psychotic symptoms have elevated rates of violent behavior."

EPIDEMIOLOGICAL CATCHMENT AREA (ECA) SURVEY (BALTIMORE, DURHAM, AND LOS ANGELES) (Swanson et al., 1990; Swanson, 1994)[3]	
Sample and Methods	**Additional Information**
• community survey of 6,911 individuals (Durham and Los Angeles) • major mental disorder = schizophrenia, bipolar disorder, and major depression • 44% male, 56% female • violence = used a weapon in a fight or more than one fight, which included "swapping blows" with someone other than spouse/partner • violence ascertained by self-report only	• 1-year prevalence of violence: 　—major mental disorders only: 7% 　—major mental disorder + substance abuse: 23% • prevalence of violence in general population: 2% • ". . . serious mental disorder by itself is quite significantly associated with violence—as shown by odds ratios in the range of about 2.4 to 3.6."

MACARTHUR VIOLENCE RISK ASSESSMENT (KANSAS CITY, PITTSBURGH, AND WORCESTER) (Steadman et al., 1998; Steadman and Silver, 1999)[4]	
Sample and Methods	**Additional Information**
• 951 individuals • 34% diagnosed with schizophrenia, bipolar disorder, or other psychoses; 40% depression, including dysthymia • 29% refusal rate, including 44% among individuals with schizophrenia • 50% dropout rate at less than 1 year • 58% male, 42% female	• 1-year prevalence of serious violence: 　—18% without substance abuse 　—31% with substance abuse • 608 total incidents of serious violence, including 6 homicides • 86% of targets were family or friends • study individuals were being con-

• serious violence = physical injury, threat or assault with weapon, sexual assault • violence ascertained by self-report, family report, and police records	tacted every 10 weeks and theoretically were being treated • marked decrease in violence from pre-hospitalization to post-hospitalization periods, showing clear effect of treatment

FOUR-STATE STUDY (CONNECTICUT, MARYLAND, NEW HAMPSHIRE, AND NORTH CAROLINA) (Swanson et al., 2002)[5]	
Sample and Methods	**Additional Information**
• 802 individuals • 83% diagnosed with schizophrenia, schizoaffective disorder, or bipolar disorder • 13% refusal rate • 65% male, 35% female • serious violence = physical injury, threat or assault with weapon, sexual assault • violence ascertained by self-report	• 1-year prevalence of serious violence: 13% • violence among males 15%; among females 11% • violence correlated with substance abuse, homelessness, and past violent victimization • almost all patients were receiving treatment, with 89% medication compliance

WORCESTER–PHILADELPHIA STUDY (Monahan et al., 2005)[6]	
Sample and Methods	**Additional Information**
• 157 individuals • 28% diagnosed with schizophrenia or bipolar disorder; 59% depression • 32% refusal rate • 54% male, 46% female • serious violence = physical injury, threat or assault with weapon, sexual assault • violence ascertained by self-report and family report	• 5-month prevalence of serious violence: 18%

CATIE STUDY (MULTIPLE SITES) (Swanson et al., 2006)[7]	
Sample and Methods	**Additional Information**
• 1,410 individuals • all diagnosed with schizophrenia • 6% refusal rate • 74% male, 26% female • serious violence = physical injury, threat or assault with weapon, sexual assault • violence ascertained by self-report and family report	• 6-month prevalence of serious violence: 4% • an additional 15% committed lesser forms of violence • males and females equally likely to commit serious violence • violence more likely in those with paranoid delusions, hallucinations, and/or grandiosity • all individuals were being treated; willingness to take medication was a requirement for inclusion in the study
FIVE-CITY STUDY (CHICAGO, DURHAM, SAN FRANCISCO, TAMPA, AND WORCESTER) (Swanson et al., 2006;[8] Elbogen et al., 2006)[9]	
Sample and Methods	**Additional Information**
• 1,011 outpatients in mental health clinics • all patients being treated, but one-third not taking medication regularly • 65% schizophrenia and bipolar disorder • refusal rates 2–13% • serious violence = assault with injury; threat/assault with lethal weapon; sexual assault • other aggressive acts = simple assault	• 6-month prevalence of serious violence: 6% • 6-month prevalence of other aggressive acts: 14% • violence rate inversely related to treatment adherence and perceived treatment need • patients who did not believe they needed treatment were 2.5 times more likely to commit acts of serious violence

APPENDIX B:

Studies from Other Countries of Homicides Committed by Individuals with Psychotic Disorders

SCOTLAND: 400 HOMICIDE OFFENDERS 1953–74 (Gillies, 1976)[1]	
Percentage of Individuals Diagnosed with Psychotic Disorders	**Additional Information**
3.0% schizophrenia 1.3% depression with psychosis 1.0% other psychoses 5.3% total	• "Schizophrenics who relapse in the community after stopping drug treatment constitute a potential hazard, but a small one." • 92% male, 8% female
GERMANY: 2,996 ATTEMPTED OR COMPLETED HOMICIDES 1955–64 (Hafner and Boker, 1982, summarized by Taylor and Gunn, 1984)[2]	
Percentage of Individuals Diagnosed with Psychotic Disorders	**Additional Information**
7.7% schizophrenia in men 6.4% schizophrenia in women	• approximately half were completed and half attempted homicides
DENMARK (COPENHAGEN): 251 HOMICIDE OFFENDERS 1959–83 (Gottlieb et al., 1987)[3]	
Percentage of Individuals Diagnosed with Psychotic Disorders	**Additional Information**
6.4% schizophrenia 1.6% "chronic paranoia"	• study included "nearly all suspects of murder"

6.8% depression with psychosis 14.8% total	• an additional 6.8% were "reactive," alcoholic, drug-induced, organic, or "other" psychoses

HONG KONG: 621 HOMICIDES 1961–71 (Wong and Singer, 1973)[4]	
Percentage of Individuals Diagnosed with Psychotic Disorders	**Additional Information**
6.2% with psychoses	• paranoid delusions common • family members disproportionately victims • female perpetrators disproportion- ately common

BARBADOS: 172 SOLVED HOMICIDES 1978–95 (Evans and Malesu, 1997)[5]	
Percentage of Individuals Diagnosed with Psychotic Disorders	**Additional Information**
9.9% schizophrenia	• 3 others diagnosed with "mood disorder"

ENGLAND (GREATER LONDON): 107 HOMICIDES 1980 (Taylor and Gunn, 1984)[6]	
Percentage of Individuals Diagnosed with Psychotic Disorders	**Additional Information**
9.3% schizophrenia 1.9% affective psychosis 11.2% total	• study included only male offenders • over 90% of the men were previ- ously known to psychiatric services, but only one-quarter were receiving treatment at the time of the homicide • the authors said their numbers were "almost certainly an underestimate of the true prevalence"

CANADA (QUEBEC): 87 HOMICIDE OFFENDERS 1988 (Coté and Hodgins, 1992)[7]	
Percentage of Individuals Diagnosed with Psychotic Disorders	**Additional Information**
10.3% schizophrenia 1.1% bipolar disorder 11.4% total	• random survey of male inmates of prisons in Quebec • diagnoses based on the illness at the time of the crime • 29% refusal rate of those invited to participate, which therefore probably did not include many with paranoid schizophrenia
NEW ZEALAND: 1,498 HOMICIDES 1970–2000 (Simpson et al., 2004)[8]	
Percentage of Individuals Diagnosed with Psychotic Disorders	**Additional Information**
3.7% schizophrenia 1.3% other psychoses 0.3% bipolar disorder 5.3% total	• diagnostic data missing on four other cases of infanticide • 71% had a prior psychiatric hospitalization, 10% in the month preceding the homicide • three-quarters of the victims were family members or partners • 67% male, 33% female
AUSTRIA: 992 HOMICIDES 1975–99 (Schanda et al., 2004, and personal communication, 2004)[9]	
Percentage of Individuals Diagnosed with Psychotic Disorders	**Additional Information**
5.8% schizophrenia 0.1% bipolar disorder 0.4% delusional disorder	• for subset for which data were available, only 6% had been on medication in the month preceding the homicide

6.3% total	• concurrent alcohol abuse a major problem • 69% male, 31% female

FINLAND: 994 HOMICIDES 1984–91 (Eronen et al., 1996a; Eronen et al., 1996b)[10]	
Percentage of Individuals Diagnosed with Psychotic Disorders	**Additional Information**
6.3% schizophrenia 2.4% other psychoses 8.7% total	• half of those with schizophrenia had paranoid subtype • alcohol abuse doubled risk of homicide • 91% male, 9% female

SWEDEN: 2,005 COMPLETED OR ATTEMPTED HOMICIDES 1988–2001 (Fazel and Grann, 2004)[11]	
Percentage of Individuals Diagnosed with Psychotic Disorders	**Additional Information**
8.9% schizophrenia 2.5% bipolar disorder 6.5% other psychoses 17.9% total	• substance abuse contributed to almost half of cases • did not include homicide perpetrators who then suicided • 92% male, 8% female

GERMANY (HESSEN): 290 COMPLETED OR ATTEMPTED HOMICIDES 1992–96 (Erb et al., 2001)[12]	
Percentage of Individuals Diagnosed with Psychotic Disorders	**Additional Information**
10.0% schizophrenia	• two-thirds (19/29) had paranoid subtype • two-thirds (18/29) had prior history of violent behavior

| | • two-thirds (18/29) had been psychi-atrically hospitalized |
| | • 86% male, 14% female |

AUSTRALIA (VICTORIA): 168 HOMICIDES 1993–95 (Wallace et al., 1998)[13]	
Percentage of Individuals Diagnosed with Psychotic Disorders	**Additional Information**
7.1% schizophrenia 1.8% affective psychosis 8.9% total	• substance abuse increased odds of homicide fourfold • only one-third had had previous contact with mental health services • 90% male, 10% female

ENGLAND AND WALES: 1,594 HOMICIDES 1996–99 (Shaw et al., 1999, 2005; Meehan et al., 2006)[14]	
Percentage of Individuals Diagnosed with Psychotic Disorders	**Additional Information**
5.3% schizophrenia	• only 20% had been in contact with mental health services in previous year • medication compliance was a major problem • 32% had a previous conviction for violent behavior • 90% male, 10% female

ENGLAND AND WALES: 2,684 HOMICIDES 1999–2003 (Appleby and Shaw, 2006)[15]	
Percentage of Individuals Diagnosed with Psychotic Disorders	**Additional Information**
5.3% schizophrenia	• 52% of those with schizophrenia had been seen by mental health services in the preceding year

	• 28% had a previous history of violence against the person killed documented in their psychiatric record
SINGAPORE: 110 HOMICIDE OFFENDERS 1997–2001 (Koh et al., 2006)[16]	
Percentage of Individuals Diagnosed with Psychotic Disorders	**Additional Information**
15.4% with psychoses	• alcohol abuse as a contributing factor was very common • 71% of those with psychoses had persecutory delusions
AUSTRALIA (NEW SOUTH WALES): 1,052 HOMICIDES 1993–2002 (Nielssen et al., 2007)[17]	
Percentage of Individuals Diagnosed with Psychotic Disorders	**Additional Information**
8.8% acute psychosis	• majority in first episode of psychosis • substance abuse was a contributing factor in the majority of cases • the majority of perpetrators believed they were in danger from the victim • "in most cases the victim was a relative or close friend" • 45% of the perpetrators had contact with mental health or social services in the two weeks before the crime

Notes

PREFACE

1. P. Duggan and T. Jackman, "Thousands mourn Fairfax detective, 'Our protector,'" *Washington Post*, May 14, 2006.
2. J. Matthews, "Son, 24, charged in mother's death," *Washington Post*, May 14, 2006.
3. E. Fuller Torrey and Sidney M. Wolfe, *Care of the Seriously Mentally Ill: A Rating of State Programs* (Washington, D.C.: Public Citizen Health Research Group, 1986); E. Fuller Torrey, Sidney M. Wolfe, and Laurie M. Flynn, *Care of the Seriously Mentally Ill: A Rating of State Programs* (Washington, D.C.: Public Citizen Health Research Group and the National Alliance for the Mentally Ill, 1988).

CHAPTER 1: INTRODUCTION: THE ORIGINS OF A DISASTER

1. F. E. Markowitz, "Psychiatric hospital capacity, homelessness, and crime and arrest rates," *Criminology* 44 (2006): 45–72.
2. Bruce Ennis, *Prisoners of Psychiatry* (New York: Harcourt Brace Jovanovich, 1972), pp. xvii, 82, 232.
3. The federal estimates are taken from the websites of the National Mental Health Information Center under the Substance Abuse and Mental Health Services Administration (www.mentalhealth.samhsa.gov) and the National Institute of Mental Health (www.nimh.nih.gov). The SSI and SSDI numbers are taken from the 2003 *Annual Statistical Supplement to the Social Security Bulletin* of the Social Security Administration (www.socialsecurity.gov/policy).
4. L. M. Davies and M. F. Drummond, "Economics and schizophrenia: The real cost," *British Journal of Psychiatry* 165, suppl. 25 (1994): 18–21.

CHAPTER 2: DEATH BY THE ROADSIDE

1. Unless otherwise noted, information and quotations from Pauline Wilkerson are taken from the author's interviews of October 6, 2004, and July 14, 2005.

2. Author interview with Garnell Wilkerson, October 6, 2004.

3. Unless otherwise noted, all quotations from Lothell Tate are taken from the transcript of her trial or appeals, accessed in the South Carolina Supreme Court library.

4. D. Suchetka, "Gaston Mental Health may investigate Tate case," *Charlotte Observer,* February 26, 1989.

5. Information on the Bobby Cannon case is taken from T. Mellnik, R. Morell, and K. Doherty, "Slain teacher's letter sought help for son," *Charlotte Observer,* December 6, 1984, pp. 1A, 10A; R. Morell, C. E. Shepard, and B. Rogers, "Bobby Cannon's life unraveled amid shattered dreams," ibid., December 7, 1984, pp. 1A, 11A; G. L. Wright, "Cannon competent to stand trial, psychiatrist says," ibid., November 9, 1985, p. 1C.

6. D. Suchetka and B. Martin, "N.C. family's final solution was murder," *Charlotte Observer,* February 27, 1989, pp. 1A, 8A.

7. Ibid.

8. Ibid.

9. See note 2 above.

CHAPTER 3: THIRTEEN MURDERS TO PREVENT AN EARTHQUAKE

1. *Santa Cruz Sentinel,* February 12, 1973, p. 1, and February 13, 1973, p. 1.

2. Donald T. Lunde and Jefferson Morgan, *The Die Song: A Journey into the Mind of a Mass Murderer* (New York: W. W. Norton, 1980), p. 220; *Santa Cruz Sentinel,* February 15, 1973, p. 1.

3. *Santa Cruz Sentinel,* February 20, 1973, p. 1.

4. Ibid.

5. Lunde and Morgan, *The Die Song,* p. 226.

6. A. H. Urmer, "An assessment of California's mental health program: Implications for mental health delivery systems," in Calvin J. Frederick, ed., *Dangerous Behavior: A Problem in Law and Mental Health* (Rockville, Md.: U.S. Department of Health, Education, and Welfare, 1978), p. 137; "New Mental Health Legislation," speech by Assemblyman Frank Lanterman, chairman, Assembly Ways and Means Subcommittee on Mental Health Services, March 23, 1968, Riverside, Calif.

7. Eugene Bardach, *The Skill Factor in Politics: Repealing the Mental Commitment Laws in California* (Berkeley: University of California Press, 1972), p. 119.

8. A. Auerbach, "The anti–mental health movement," *American Journal of Psychiatry* 120 (1963):105–12. This material is also taken from letters from Ms. Gene Birkeland to me, dated February 4, 1994, and February 11, 2000; and D. Robinson, "Conspiracy USA," *Look,* January 26, 1965, pp. 30–32.

9. R. Schmuck and M. Chesler, "Superpatriot opposition to community mental health programs," *Community Mental Health Journal* 3 (1967): 382–88.

10. N. Petris, "The Lanterman-Petris-Short Act with a focus upon dangerousness," in Frederick, ed., *Dangerous Behavior,* p. 102.

11. N. Petris, "New approaches to mental health in the California Legislature," in

Calvin J. Frederick, ed., *The Future of Psychotherapy* (Boston: Little, Brown, 1969), pp. 361–78.

12. Bardach, *The Skill Factor*, pp. 114, 126.

13. Lanterman, "New Mental Health Legislation."

14. Lunde and Morgan, *The Die Song*, p. 309.

15. Ibid., p. 229.

16. Ibid., p. 141.

17. *Santa Cruz Sentinel*, August 7, 1973, p. 1, and August 8, 1973, p. 1; Lunde and Morgan, *The Die Song*, pp. 182, 296.

18. Lunde and Morgan, *The Die Song*, p. 237.

19. *Santa Cruz Sentinel*, August 3, 1973, p. 1.

20. Lunde and Morgan, *The Die Song*, p. 239.

21. Ibid., p. 240.

22. *Santa Cruz Sentinel*, August 14, 1973, p. 2; Lunde and Morgan, *The Die Song*, p. 247.

23. *Santa Cruz Sentinel*, August 15, 1973, p. 2.

24. Lunde and Morgan, *The Die Song*, pp. 277.

25. Ibid., p. 277, 278.

26. *Santa Cruz Sentinel*, August 20, 1973, p. 2.

27. "Jury foreman rips governor," *Santa Cruz Sentinel*, August 22, 1973, p. 1.

CHAPTER 4: "THE ODDS ARE STILL IN SOCIETY'S FAVOR"

1. S. P. Segal, M. A. Watson, S. M. Goldfinger, et al., "Civil commitment in the psychiatric emergency room: II. Mental disorder indicators and three dangerousness criteria," *Archives of General Psychiatry* 45 (1988): 753–58.

2. Arnold A. Rogow, *The Psychiatrists* (New York: G. P. Putnam's Sons, 1970), p. 126; Martin L. Gross, *The Psychological Society: A Critical Analysis of Psychiatry, Psychotherapy, Psychoanalysis, and the Psychological Revolution* (New York: Random House, 1978), p. 62.

3. K. Horak, "In 'perfect American family,' tragedy hits twice in 2 years," *Washington Post*, March 27, 1983, A10.

4. E. Fuller Torrey, *Nowhere to Go: The Tragic Odyssey of the Homeless Mentally Ill* (New York: Harper and Row, 1988), p. 197.

5. A. H. Urmer, "An assessment of California's mental health program: Implications for mental health delivery systems," in Calvin J. Frederick, ed., *Dangerous Behavior: A Problem in Law and Mental Health* (Rockville, Md.: Department of Health, Education, and Welfare, 1978), pp. 137–51; A. H. Urmer, "Implications of California's new mental health law," *American Journal of Psychiatry* 132 (1975): 251–54.

6. U. Aviram and S. P. Segal, "Exclusion of the mentally ill," *Archives of General Psychiatry* 29 (1973): 126–31.

7. M. F. Abramson, "The criminalization of mentally disordered behavior: Possible side-effect of a new mental health law," *Hospital and Community Psychiatry* 23 (1972): 101–5.

8. " 'Murder capital of the world': Three grisly mass-murder sprees plunged the county into terror," *Santa Cruz Sentinel Online Edition*, http://www.santacruzsentinel .com/extra/century/73/; Donald T. Lunde, *Murder and Madness* (Stanford, Calif.: Stanford Alumni Association, 1975), p. 51.

9. This and other quotations are from the Hearings of the Select Committee on Proposed Phaseout of State Hospital Services, May 18 to October 10, 1973, California State Archives.

10. H. R. Lamb and V. Goertzel, "Discharged mental patients—Are they really in the community?" *Archives of General Psychiatry* 24 (1971): 29–34; H. R. Lamb and V. Goertzel, "The demise of the state hospital—A premature obituary?" *Archives of General Psychiatry* 26 (1972): 489–95; Aviram and Segal, "Exclusion of the mentally ill"; M. Greenblatt and E. Glazier, "The phasing out of mental hospitals in the United States," *American Journal of Psychiatry* 132 (1975): 1135–39.

11. J. M. Stubblebine and J. B. Decker, "Are urban mental health centers worth it?" *American Journal of Psychiatry* 127 (1971): 908–12; J. M. Stubblebine and J. B. Decker, "Are urban mental health centers worth it? Part II," *American Journal of Psychiatry* 128 (1971): 480–83.

12. Albert H. Urmer, *A Study of California's New Mental Health Law* (Chatsworth, Calif.: ENKI Research Institute, 1971); A. R. Link and L. McMaster, CSEA legal brief presented in the California Superior Court, 1972; Abramson, "The criminalization of mentally disordered behavior"; *The Burden of the Mentally Disordered on Law Enforcement* (Chatsworth, Calif.: ENKI Research Institute, 1973.

13. Abramson, "The criminalization of mentally disordered behavior."

14. J. Chase, "Where have all the patients gone?" *Human Behavior* 2 (1973): 14–21; Lunde, *Murder and Madness*, p. 55.

15. L. Sosowsky, "Crime and violence among mental patients reconsidered in view of the new legal relationship between the state and the mentally ill," *American Journal of Psychiatry* 135 (1978): 33–42. The Department of Mental Health study was entitled "Violent Crime Offenders Study" and dated October 12, 1973. Sosowsky noted that he had "apparently received one of the few copies distributed." In September 2005, I attempted to locate a copy of the study in the California State Archives but was unable to do so.

16. Hearings of the Select Committee on Proposed Phaseout of State Hospital Services, May 18 to October 10, 1973, California State Archives. Also quoted in Chase, "Where have all the patients gone?"

17. R. R. Parlour, "The reorganization of the California Department of Mental Hygiene," *American Journal of Psychiatry* 128 (1972): 1388–94.

18. "Homeless mentally ill: States take action," *American Medical News*, September 20, 1985, pp. 2, 23; H. R. Lamb, "Deinstitutionalization at the crossroads," *Hospital and Community Psychiatry* 39 (1988): 941–45.

19. R. K. Farr, *The Homeless Mentally Ill and the Los Angeles Skid Row Mental Health Project* (Los Angeles County: Department of Mental Health, 1985).

20. L. Gelberg and L. S. Linn, "Social and physical health of homeless adults previously treated for mental health problems," *Hospital and Community Psychiatry* 39

(1988): 510–16; H. R. Lamb and D. M. Lamb, "Factors contributing to homelessness among the chronically and severely mentally ill," ibid., 41 (1990): 301–5.

21. C. G. Craddock, "Plight of the mentally ill homeless in L.A." (letter), *Los Angeles Times*, February 8, 1986, p. 15.

22. L. Ludlow, "Over the edge and on the streets: Mentally ill homeless near crisis in S.F.," *San Francisco Chronicle*, December 27, 1987, A1, A16; letter to the author, August 1992; P. Matier and A. Ross, "Agnos draws fire on city shelters for the homeless," *San Francisco Examiner*, May 12, 1991, A1, A14.

23. M. Janofsky, "Mild and merciful San Francisco a magnet for the homeless," *New York Times*, August 16, 1998, p. 20; M Curtius, "San Francisco mayor says city's homeless problem may not be solvable," *Washington Post*, October 13, 1996, A12; B. Mandel, "The homeless are a cancer on city's soul," *San Francisco Examiner*, January 14, 1990, B3; E. Nieves, "Fed up, Berkeley begins crackdown on homeless," *New York Times*, November 3, 1998, A19.

24. H. R. Lamb and R. W. Grant, "The mentally ill in an urban county jail," *Archives of General Psychiatry* 39 (1982): 17–22; H. R. Lamb and R. W. Grant, "Mentally ill women in a county jail," ibid., 40 (1983): 363–68; H. R. Lamb, R. Schock, P. W. Chen, et al., "Psychiatric needs in local jails: Emergency issues," *American Journal of Psychiatry* 141 (1984): 774–77; H. R. Lamb, "Incompetency to stand trial," *Archives of General Psychiatry* 44 (1987): 754–58; G. E. Whitmer, "From hospitals to jails," *American Journal of Orthopsychiatry* 50 (1980): 65–75.

25. "Homelessness in San Francisco" (San Francisco: Caduceus Outreach Services, 1995); S. Robitaille, "Statistics paint picture of a system in distress," (San Jose) *Mercury News*, February 16, 1992; "Mental health cuts unlock doors to new treatments," *Sacramento Bee*, October 4, 1994, p. 10; J. A. Santoro, "Stop using jails as mental hospitals," *Los Angeles Times*, August 29, 1998; "Trapped inside" (news transcript), KNBC 4, Los Angeles, May 8, 2003.

26. T. Daunt, "Mentally ill at risk in county jails, study says," *Los Angeles Times*, March 30, 1997, A1.

27. M. Collet, "The crime of mental health," (Pleasanton, Calif.) *Valley Times*, December 15, 1981; C. LeDuff, "A jail tour in Los Angeles offers a peek into 5 killings behind bars," *New York Times*, May 23, 2004, p. 14; H. Tobar, "County OKs payment in jail beating," *Los Angeles Times*, June 9, 1992.

28. R. Jemelka, "The mentally ill in local jails," in H. J. Steadman, ed., *Jail Diversion for the Mentally Ill* (Washington, D.C.: U.S. Department of Justice, National Institute of Corrections, 1990), p. 43, citing a study by L. LeBrun.

29. M. J. O'Sullivan, "Criminializing the mentally ill," *America* 166 (1992): 8–13; T. Saavedra, "Mentally ill winding up in jails," *Orange County Register*, March 7, 1999.

30. J. R. Husted, R. A. Charter and B. Perrou, "California law enforcement agencies and the mentally ill offender," *Bulletin of the American Academy of Psychiatry and the Law* 23 (1995): 315–29; Chase, "Where have all the patients gone?"; H. Tobar, "When jail is a mental institution," *Los Angeles Times*, August 25–26, 1991.

31. *Los Angeles Times*, July 28, 2001; ibid., January 29, 2002; data from a Ventura

County Grand Jury Report, "Fatal Shootings in Ventura County by Law Enforcement Officers, 1992–2001," Office of the Ventura County District Attorney.

32. Sosowsky, "Crime and violence among mental patients reconsidered"; L. Sosowsky, "Explaining the increased arrest rate among mental patients: A cautionary note," *American Journal of Psychiatry* 137 (1980): 1602–5. The study was publicly released in 1974 and subsequently published in 1978 and 1980.

33. P. Weisser, "A blast at mental care," *San Francisco Chronicle*, September 20, 1974, p. 4.

34. S. J. Sansweet, "Release of mentally ill into communities stirs much debate, and fear," *Wall Street Journal*, August 19, 1976; Sosowsky, "Crime and violence among mental patients reconsidered"; Sosowsky, "Explaining the increased arrest rate among mental patients."

35. These and many other examples can be accessed on the website of the Treatment Advocacy Center, www.treatmentadvocacycenter.org; click on preventable tragedies, then on California.

36. *Sacramento Bee*, June 8, 2001.

37. D. P. Folsom, W. Hawthorne, L. Lindamer, et al., "Prevalence and risk factors for homelessness and utilization of mental health services among 10,340 patients with serious mental illness in a large public mental health system," *American Journal of Psychiatry* 162 (2005): 370–76.

38. S. Lopez, "Now comes the heavy lifting," *Los Angeles Times*, October 23, 2005; L. Romney and S. Gold, "Gov. seeks to cut mental services for homeless," ibid., July 14, 2007.

39. P. Teetor, "Prelude to a death," *Los Angeles Times*, May 5, 2002; C. Quanbeck, M. Frye and L. Altshuler, "Mania and the law in California: Understanding the criminalization of the mentally ill," *American Journal of Psychiatry* 160 (2003): 1245–50.

40. J. Johnson, "Jail suicides reach record pace in state," *Los Angeles Times*, June 16, 2002; J. Dearen, "Mental patients languish in jails," *Oakland Tribune*, September 22, 2005.

41. L. Udesky, "Court takes over California's prison health system," *Lancet* 366 (2005): 796–97; D. Morain and J. Warren, "Battle looms over prison spending in state budget," *Los Angeles Times*, January 22, 2003.

42. J. Robertson, "Mother pleads innocent to killing sons," Associated Press, October 21, 2005; C. Marshall, "Woman charged in deaths of her 3 children," *New York Times*, October 21, 2005.

43. R. C. Archibold, "Death toll climbs to 8 in California postal plant rampage," *New York Times*, February 2, 2006.

44. L. Parrilla and S. Curran, "Paranoic, homelessness gripped Pismo gunman," *Mercury News*, March 17, 2006.

45. S. Smith, "Experts: Mentally ill face criminal stigma," *Stockton Record*, November 24, 2005.

46. "Fatal Shootings in Ventura County by Law Enforcement Officers, 1992–2001," Report of a Ventura County Grand Jury, 2001–2002.

47. D. A. Treffert, "It took awhile" (editorial), *Wisconsin Psychiatrist*, Winter 2001.

48. A. Marroquin, "Inland man drove truck into Capitol," (Riverside) *Press-Enterprise*, January 18, 2001; C. Sanders, "Bowers no stranger to the local media," ibid., January 24, 2001; B. C. Bird, "What goes around comes around," *www.geocities.com/ CapitolHill/Parliament/2398/bowers.html?200617*, accessed September 4, 2006.

49. The Lewin Group, *Costs of Serving Homeless Individuals in Nine Cities* (chart book prepared for the Corporation for Supportive Housing), November 18, 2004.

CHAPTER 5: THE KILLING OF THREE DEVILS

1. The account of the Bryan Stanley murders and subsequent events was taken from the following articles in the *La Crosse Tribune*: G. Achterberg, February 8, 1985; R. Erikson, February 6, 2005, and P. Sloth, February 6, 2005; M. Hanson and T. Rindfleisch, October 30, 1985; Rindfleisch, February 8, 1985; B. McClellan, February 11, 1985; Hanson, February 13, 1985; G. Hollnagel, April 7, 1985; Rindfleisch, October 29, 1985; Rindfleisch, February 11, 1985; Rindfleisch, October 31, 1985; Rindfleisch, February 6, 2005; K. Teachout, February 24, 1985; Hollnagel, February 11, 1985; Hanson, June 4, 1985; and Rindfleisch, October 31, 1985; and from interview notes of Dr. Frederick Fosdal, July 1, 1985, in the Bryan Stanley file, La Crosse County Courthouse.

2. Robert D. Miller, letter to the judge, La Crosse County Circuit Court, May 2, 1985, in the Bryan Stanley file, La Crosse County Courthouse.

3. Civil Action Case No. 71-C-602, *Lessard v. Schmidt*, Stipulation of Facts, Appendix I, Testimony of Officer James D. Mejchar, March 30, 1972.

4. Telephone interviews with Robert H. Blondis, January 14, 2004, and July 29, 2004. The Supreme Court case was *Shelton v. Tucker*, 364 U.S. 479 (1960).

5. *Lessard v. Schmidt,* 349 F. Supp. 1078 (E. D. Wis. 1972); Alexander D. Brooks, "Notes on Defining the 'Dangerousness' of the Mentally Ill," in Calvin J. Frederick, ed., *Dangerous Behavior: A Problem in Law and Mental Health* (Rockville, Md.: U.S. Department of Health, Education, and Welfare, 1978).

6. *Lessard v. Schmidt,* quoting Livermore et al., *On the Justifications for Civil Commitment,* 117 Pa. L. Rev. 75, 80 (1968); Bruce Ennis, *Prisoners of Psychiatry: Mental Patients, Psychiatrists, and Law* (New York: Harcourt Brace Jovanovich, 1972), p. 232; statement of Bruce J. Ennis, Hearings on the Constitutional Rights of the Mentally Ill, Subcommittee on Constitutional Rights, Committee on the Judiciary, U.S. Senate, November 4, 5, 12, 13, 18, and 19, 273 (1969).

7. Ennis, Senate Hearings, op cit.; Thomas Szasz, *Law, Liberty, and Psychiatry* (New York: Collier Books, 1968), p. 240 (originally published in 1963); *Lessard v. Schmidt.*

8. Alan A. Stone, *Mental Health and Law: A System in Transition* (New York: Jason Aronson, 1976); D. A. Treffert, "The obviously ill patient in need of treatment: A fourth standard for civil commitment," *Hospital and Community Psychiatry* 36 (1985): 259–64.

CHAPTER 6: THE SAD LEGACY OF MS. LESSARD

1. John Locke, *Two Treatises of Government*, Peter Laslett, ed. (New York: Mentor Books, 1965), pp. 348–52 (originally published in London, circa 1690); M. J. Remington, "*Lessard v. Schmidt* and its implications for involuntary civil commitment in Wisconsin," *Marquette Law Review* 57 (1973): 65–101.

2. M. Zahn and D. Patrinos, "Criminal complaint filed so daughter can get help," *Milwaukee Sentinel*, August 18, 1981; M. Kissinger, "Does law help or hurt mentally ill?" *Milwaukee Journal*, June 17, 1984.

3. D. Patrinos and M. Zahn, "Man moves in, out of system," *Milwaukee Sentinel*, August 19, 1981.

4. T. K. Zander, "Civil commitment in Wisconsin: The impact of *Lessard v. Schmidt*," *Wisconsin Law Review* 19 (1976): 503–63; M. Kissinger, "Does law help or hurt mentally ill?"; M. Kissinger, "Balancing the thin edge of recovery," *Milwaukee Journal Sentinel*, September 16, 2000.

5. H. L. Mitternight, "Number of homeless is straining shelters," *Milwaukee Journal*, November 26, 1982; M. I. Blackwell, "Fight for homeless probes roots," ibid., December 22, 1983; M. I. Blackwell, "Homeless mentally ill: Problem is growing, showing," ibid., November 22, 1984; T. Roets, ibid., November 9, 1984; M. Ward, Street people: Who are they and why are they there?" ibid., February 5, 1986; M. Kissinger, "Teacher's case opened door for mentally ill," *Milwaukee Journal Sentinel*, August 27, 2000.

6. J. Manning, "Legal system seen as hurting mentally ill," *Milwaukee Sentinel*, May 3, 1991, p. 5; "On the street," *Milwaukee Journal*, February 21, 1988; M. Kissinger, "Lost on the streets," *Milwaukee Journal Sentinel*, August 26, 2000; M. Kissinger, "Teacher's case opened door for mentally ill;" D. Patrinos and M. Zahn, "Falling through the cracks, troubled minds lack care," *Milwaukee Sentinel*, August 20, 1981.

7. M. Kupper, "Ex-Packer wants back in the game of life," *Milwaukee Journal*, December 14, 1983.

8. L. Penrose, "Mental disease and crime: Outline of a comparative study of European statistics," *British Journal of Psychiatry* 18 (1938): 1–15.

9. D. Treffert, "Legal rites: Criminalizing the mentally ill," *Hillside Journal of Clinical Psychiatry* 3 (1982): 123–37.

10. M. Zahn, "Mentally ill given a cell instead of proper care," *Milwaukee Sentinel*, August 17, 1981; Patrinos and Zahn, "Falling through the cracks."

11. M. Kissinger, "Promise of care made but broken," *Milwaukee Journal Sentinel*, March 19, 2006; Zahn, Mentally ill given a cell"; Patrinos and Zahn, "Falling through the cracks."

12. Zahn, "Mentally ill given a cell"; Patrinos and Zahn, "Falling through the cracks."

13. M. Kissinger, "Trading one locked door for another," *Milwaukee Journal Sentinel*, September 9, 2000; P. Marley, "Thousands with mental illness still lack proper care in prison," ibid., September 11, 2004.

14. R. Magney, "County group examining jail, mental illness issues," *La Crosse Tribune*,

March 5, 2001; R. Magney, "Is the jail doing enough," ibid., November 21, 2002; B. Bloom, "Filled to capacity," ibid., May 26, 2002.

15. Kissinger, "Trading one locked door for another."

16. Ibid.

17. Ibid.

18. Ibid.; "Inmate denied MH treatment wins record settlement," *Psychiatric News*, May 7, 1999.

19. D. A. Treffert, "Dying with one's rights on" (letter), *Journal of the American Medical Association* 224 (1973): 1649; D. A. Treffert, "Dying with their rights on," *Prism*, 1974; D. A. Treffert, "The MacArthur Coercion Studies: A Wisconsin perspective," *Marquette Law Review* 82 (1999): 759–85.

20. Information in vignettes is taken from the following sources: (Marquardt) *Duluth News Tribune*, February 8, 2005; (Lubeck) WKMG-TV CBS 6, November 11, 2004.

21. Information in vignettes is taken from the following sources: (Blucher) *Duluth News Tribune*, September 7, 2004, *Milwaukee Journal Sentinel*, September 7, 2004, MSNBC.com, November 22, 2004, *Milwaukee Journal Sentinel*, November 24, 2004, ibid., November 25, 2004; (Yang) ibid., January 28, 2005, and February 17, 2005.

22. Information in vignettes is taken from the following sources: (Kartman) Associated Press, September 17 and 29, 1998; (fifty-one-year-old man) *Milwaukee Journal Sentinel*, July 7, 1999.

23. Information in vignettes is taken from the following sources: (Blodgett) Associated Press, March 23, 1999; (fifty-four-year-old woman) ibid., January 19, 2001.

24. Information in vignettes is taken from the following sources: (Humphrey) Associated Press, April 5, 1999; (Bradley) *Green Bay Press Gazette*, July 14, 2004.

25. Information in vignettes is taken from the following sources: (Crispin) *La Crosse Tribune*, July 22, 2003; (Nash) *Milwaukee Journal Sentinel*, July 31, 2003; (Graf) *Sussex Sun*, June 11, 2003; (Dukart) *Marshfield News-Herald*, September 13, 2003; (Hirte) WTMJ-TV NBC 4, February 1, 2005, *Oshkosh Northwestern*, February 4, 2005; (Addy) WDJT-TV, January 6, 2004, *Milwaukee Journal Sentinel*, December 19, 2003; (O'Neal) (Madison, Wisc.) *Capital Times*, June 27, 2003, August 2, 2003, September 20, 2003, October 17, 2003, February 23, 2004, February 26, 2004; (Dykas) *Milwaukee Journal Sentinel*, September 13, 2003, *Gazette Extra*, April 30, 2004; (Larson) *Sheboygan Press*, May 23, 2003, May 28, 2003, September 9, 2003, December 30, 2003, February 19, 2004.

26. The literature on PACT programs is voluminous. Some of the more pertinent studies include L. I. Stein and M. A. Test, "Alternative to mental hospital treatment: I. Conceptual model, treatment program, and clinical evaluation," *Archives of General Psychiatry* 37 (1980): 392–97; B. A. Weisbrod, M. A. Test, and L. I. Stein, "Alternative to mental hospital treatment: II. Economic benefit-cost analysis," ibid., 400–405; L. Dixon, P. Weiden, M. Torres, et al., "Assertive community treatment and medication compliance in the homeless mentally ill," *American Journal of Psychiatry* 154 (1997): 1302–4; N. Wolff, T. W. Helminiak, and R. J. Diamond,

"Estimated societal costs of assertive community mental health care," *Psychiatric Services* 46 (1995): 898–906; E. F. Torrey, "Continuous treatment teams in the care of the chronic mentally ill," *Hospital and Community Psychiatry* 37 (1986): 1243–47; A. F. Lehman, L. B. Dixon, E. Kernan, et al., "A randomized trial of assertive community treatment for homeless persons with severe mental illness," *Archives of General Psychiatry* 54 (1997): 1038–43; B. J. Burns and A. B. Santos, "Assertive community treatment: An update of randomized trials," *Psychiatric Services* 46 (1995): 669–75; G. B. Teague, R. E. Drake, and T. H. Ackerson, "Evaluating use of continuous treatment teams for persons with mental illness and substance abuse," ibid., 689–95; K. S. Thompson, E. E. H. Griffith and P. J. Leaf, "A historical review of the Madison Model of community care," *Hospital and Community Psychiatry* 41 (1990): 625–32.

27. D. Mell, "Cardinal Hotel eyed for destitute," *Wisconsin State Journal*, May 26, 1982; "Putting order in bums' lives," *Capital Times*, June 28, 1984; D. Medaris, "Housing the homeless," *Isthmus*, January 11, 1985; B. Mulhern, "Madison area seeks ways to cope with homelessness," *Capital Times*, February 20, 1988.

28. M. A. Test, W. H. Knoedler, D. J. Allness, et al., "Young adults with schizophrenic disorders in the community" (paper presented at the annual meeting of the American Psychiatric Association, Los Angeles, Calif., May 5–11, 1984); D. Allegretti, "Study: Mentally ill often wrongly jailed," *Capital Times*, April 25, 1985; L. Tiajoloff, "Here's the inside story of mental health's biggest conundrum," *Isthmus*, December 13, 1985.

29. T. L. Kuhlman, "Unavoidable tragedies in Madison, Wisconsin: A third view," *Hospital and Community Psychiatry* 43 (1992): 72–3; D. Blaska, "Suspect changed from 'nice guy' to 'weird,' " *Capital Times*, January 16, 1989.

30. M. Stamler, "Zoo's bear had to die, but his death still hurts," *Capital Times*, March 14, 1988, p. 1; "Bear's hide saved, body sent to UW," ibid., March 15, 1988, p. 1; "Troubled man's life is still of value" (editorial), ibid., March 16, 1988, p. 14; "Zoo tragedy needs long-term cure" (editorial), ibid., March 21, 1988.

31. B. Mulhern, "Jailing mentally ill poses dilemma," *Capital Times*, March 19, 1988; P. Wendling, "Is more jail space the best solution?" ibid., January 15, 1988.

32. G. J. Maier, "The tragedies of Madison"; T. L. Kuhlman, "Unavoidable tragedies in Madison, Wisconsin"; R. J. Diamond, "Coercion and tenacious treatment in the community: Applications to the real world," in Deborah L. Dennis and John Monahan, eds., *Coercion and Aggressive Community Treatment: A New Frontier in Mental Health Law* (New York: Plenum Press, 1996), pp. 51–72.

33. Tiajoloff, "Here's the inside story."

34. D. Greenley, "The tragedies of Madison" (letter), *Hospital and Community Psychiatry* 43 (1992): 402–3; D. Greenley, "Advocacy in Wisconsin" (letter), ibid., 40 (1989): 1198–99; N. Jacobson and D. Greenley, "What is recovery?: A conceptual model and explication," *Psychiatric Services* 52 (2001): 482–85; Maier, "The tragedies in Madison."

35. J. Richgels and M. Stone, "Homeless people sleep in city hall at night," *Capital Times*, May 7, 1991; B. Mulern, "Everyone's problem, no one's priority," ibid.,

December 15–18, 1990; A. Weier, "Mental cases jam the jail," ibid., August 3, 1998.

36. J. Kaplan, G. Papajohn, and E. Zorn, *Murder of Innocence: The Tragic Life and Final Rampage of Laurie Dann* (New York: Warner Books, 1990), pp. 190–91, 204; B. Peterson, "Tainted food tied to school rampage," *Washington Post*, May 22, 1988, p. A3; E. Culotta, "Rights of the mentally ill," *Milwaukee Journal*, May 23, 1988.

37. Information in vignettes is taken from the following sources: (Devoe) "Man accused of beating woman with a stapler," *New York Times*, April 13, 1997, p. 15, *Capital Times*, September 11, 1997; (Grady) *Wisconsin State Journal*, January 6, 1998, *Capital Times*, January 6, 1998; (Amara) Associated Press, June 4, 1998, and October 7, 1999, *Wisconsin State Journal*, June 4, 1998, *Capital Times*, August 20, 1998, *Milwaukee Journal Sentinel*, September 30, 1998; (Orlik) *Telegraph Herald*, February 11, 1999, p. 11; (Gettridge) *Capital Times*, September 17, 1998.

38. D. A. Treffert, "The obviously ill patient in need of treatment: A fourth standard for civil commitment," *Hospital and Community Psychiatry* 36 (1985): 259–64.

39. M. Hanson, "Aftermath of a tragedy: The Stanleys: Hurt won't end," *La Crosse Tribune*, February 13, 1985; S. Miller and T. Rindfleisch, "Suspect's kin testifies for change in law," ibid., September 11, 1985.

40. G. Hollnagel, "Mom seeks 5th rule for commitment," *La Crosse Tribune*, October 13, 1990, p. A10; Memorandum from David Goodrick to Michael J. Moore, Division of Community Services, August 10, 1984.

41. Letters from Thomas Zander to the author, June 14, 2006, and July 3, 2006; Zander, "Civil commitment in Wisconsin: The impact of *Lessard v. Schmidt*."

42. M. Zahn and D. Patrinos, "2 sides see behavior as choice or disease," *Milwaukee Sentinel*, August 18, 1981; N. Jacobson and D. Greenley, "A conceptual model of recovery" (letter), *Psychiatric Services* 52 (2001): 688; D. Greenley, "Face off," *Wisconsin Counties*, June 1991, pp. 25, 37.

43. D. A. Treffert, "Update on the fifth standard," *Wisconsin Psychiatrist*, Spring 2000, pp. 24–25, and Treffert, personal communication, April 14, 2006.

44. E. Bender, "Wisconsin court rejects attempt to narrow commitment law," *Psychiatric News*, December 20, 2002.

45. D. Umhoefer, "Wrestling with the shadows," *Milwaukee Journal Sentinel*, September 2, 2000.

46. M. Kissinger, "Mentally ill suffer deadly neglect," *Milwaukee Journal Sentinel*, March 18, 2006; M. Kissinger, "Promise of care."

47. Ibid.

48. T. Rindfleisch, "Hammes kin says Stanley 'got off,' " *La Crosse Tribune*, November 1, 1985.

49. Letter from Bryan Stanley to Judge Pappas, November 15, 1985, in the court records of Bryan Stanley, case 85–79, La Crosse County Courthouse; T. Rindfleisch, "Mental health is her mission," *La Crosse Tribune*, October 22, 1986; "Stanley wants to be understood," ibid., February 7, 1989.

50. Record of 1999 hearings to determine whether Bryan Stanley should be released

from Mendota State Hospital, in his court records, case 85–79, La Crosse County Courthouse.

51. Unless otherwise noted, the information in this section came from my personal interview with Ms. Lessard on March 3, 2006, and from a previous telephone interview with her on January 26, 2004.

52. *Lessard v. State of Wisconsin*, 449 F. Supp. 914 and 462 F. Supp. 338.

53. Telephone interviews with Judge Myron L. Gordon, December 11, 2003, and January 14, 2004.

54. Court records on Alberta Lessard were obtained from the Milwaukee County Clerk of Circuit Court.

55. M. Kissinger, "What can be done?" *Milwaukee Journal Sentinel*, March 20, 2006.

CHAPTER 7: GOD DOES NOT TAKE MEDICATION

1. Thomas Dekker, *The Honest Whore* (1604) part 1, act 4, scene 3; "Confinement of the insane," *American Law Review* 3 (1869): 215; Emil Kraepelin, *Manic-Depressive Insanity and Paranoia* (North Stratford, N.H.: Ayer, 2002), p. 22, originally published in 1921); H. G. Woodley, *Certified: An Autobiographical Study* (London: Victor Gollancz, 1947), p. 89.

2. X. F. Amador, M. Flaum, N. C. Andreasen, et al., "Awareness of illness in schizophrenia and schizoaffective and mood disorders," *Archives of General Psychiatry* 51 (1994): 826–36; S. N. Ghaemi and K. J. Rosenquist, "Is insight in mania state-dependent?: A meta-analysis," *Journal of Nervous and Mental Disease* 192 (2004): 771–75.

3. These and other examples are found in M. Nathanson, P. S. Bergman, and G. G. Gordon, "Denial of illness: Its occurrence in one hundred consecutive cases of hemiplegia," *Archives of Neurology and Psychiatry* 68 (1952): 380–87; Edwin A. Weinstein and Robert L. Kahn, *Denial of Illness: Symbolic and Physiological Aspects* (Springfield, Ill.: Charles C. Thomas, 1955), p. 20; E. Bisiach and G. Feminiani, "Anosognosia related to hemiplegia and hemianopia," in G. P. Prigatano and D. L. Schacter, eds., *Awareness of Deficit after Brain Injury: Clinical and Theoretical Issues* (New York: Oxford University Press, 1991), pp. 32–33; J. Shreeve, "The brain that misplaced its body," *Discover* magazine, May 1, 1995.

4. Antonio R. Damasio, *Descartes' Error: Emotion, Reason, and the Human Brain* (New York: Avon Books, 1994), p. 64; Oliver Sacks, *The Man Who Mistook His Wife for a Hat and Other Clinical Tales* (New York: Harper Perennial, 1990), p. 5.

5. S. Kotler-Cope and C. J. Camp, "Anosognosia in Alzheimer disease," *Alzheimer Disease and Associated Disorders* 9 (1995): 52–56; R. Migliorelli, A. Tesón, L. Sabe, et al., "Anosognosia in Alzheimer's disease: A study of associated factors," *Journal of Neuropsychiatry and Clinical Neurosciences* 7 (1995): 338–44.

6. M. Roberts, "Tracy Moore finds help to control her schizophrenia, allowing her to use her singing talents for a try at stardom on 'American Idol,' " *Oregonian*, January 23, 2004; E. F. Torrey, *Surviving Schizophrenia: A Manual for Families, Patients, and Providers,* 5th ed. (New York: HarperCollins, 2006), p. 50.

7. J. Cutting, "Study of anosognosia," *Journal of Neurology, Neurosurgery, and Psychiatry*

41 (1978): 548–55; B. R. Reed, W. J. Jagust, and L. Coulter, "Anosognosia in Alzheimer's disease: Relationships to depression, cognitive function, and cerebral perfusion," *Journal of Clinical and Experimental Neuropsychology* 15 (1993): 231–44; E. A. Weinstein, "Anosognosia and denial of illness," in Prigatano and Schacter, *Awareness of Deficit after Brain Injury*, pp. 240–57.

8. F. Larøi, M. Fannemel, U. Rønneberg, et al., "Unawareness in chronic schizophrenia and its relationship to structural brain measures and neuropsychological tests," *Psychiatry Research: Neuroimaging* 100 (2000): 49–58; M. U. Shad, S. Muddasani, K. Prasad, et al., "Insight and prefrontal cortex in first-episode schizophrenia," *NeuroImage* 22 (2004): 1315–20; L. A. Flashman, T. W. McAllister, S. C. Johnson, et al., "Specific frontal lobe subregions correlated with unawareness of illness in schizophrenia: A preliminary study," *Journal of Neuropsychiatry and Clinical Neurosciences* 13 (2001): 255–57; P. Nopoulos, J. Heath, and N. C. Andreasen, "The neurobiology of insight in schizophrenia: Relationship of awareness to frontal and parietal brain regions" (abstract), *Schizophrenia Bulletin* 33 (2007): 350; M. A. Cooke, A. Sapara, I. Aasen, et al., "Smaller left inferior frontal lobe associated with poorer insight into illness in schizophrenia" (abstract), *Schizophrenia Research* 81 (2006): 158; M. U. Shad, S. Muddasani, B. Thomas, et al., "Insight and parietal cortical volume in schizophrenia" (abstract), *Schizophrenia Bulletin* 33 (2007): 355; L. A. Flashman, T. W. McAllister, N. C. Andreasen, et al., "Smaller brain size associated with unawareness of illness in patients with schizophrenia," *American Journal of Psychiatry* 157 (2000): 1167–69.

9. J. A. Cramer and R. Rosenheck, "Compliance with medication regimens for mental and physical disorders," *Psychiatric Services* 49 (1998): 196–201; J. P. Lacro, L. B. Dunn, C. R. Dolder, et al., "Prevalence of and risk factors for medication nonadherence in patients with schizophrenia: A comprehensive review of recent literature," *Journal of Clinical Psychiatry* 63 (2002): 892–909; J. P. McEvoy, "The relationship between insight into psychosis and compliance with medication," in Xavier F. Amador and Anthony S. David, eds., *Insight and Psychosis*, 2nd ed. (New York: Oxford University Press, 2004), pp. 335–50; P. E. Keck, S. L. McElroy, S. M. Strakowski, et al., "Compliance with maintenance treatment in bipolar disorder," *Psychopharmacology Bulletin* 33 (1997): 87–91; F. Colom, E. Vieta, A. Martínez-Arán, et al., "Clinical factors associated with treatment noncompliance in euthymic bipolar patients," *Journal of Clinical Psychiatry* 61 (2000): 549–55; M. Sajatovic, M. S. Bauer, A. M. Kilbourne, et al., "Self-reported medication treatment adherence among veterans with bipolar disorder," *Psychiatric Services* 57 (2006): 56–62.

10. C. M. Smith, D. Barzman, and C. A. Pristach, "Effect of patient and family insight on compliance of schizophrenic patients," *Journal of Clinical Pharmacology* 37 (1997): 147–54; M. Olfson, S. C. Marcus, J. Wilk, et al., "Awareness of illness and nonadherence to antipsychotic medications among persons with schizophrenia," *Psychiatric Services* 57 (2006): 205–11.

11. D. W. Heinrichs, B. P. Cohen, and W. T. Carpenter Jr., "Early insight and the management of schizophrenic decompensation," *Journal of Nervous and Mental Disease* 173 (1985): 133–38; P. J. Weiden, C. Kozma, A. Grogg, et al., "Partial compliance

and risk of rehospitalization among California Medicare patients with schizophrenia," *Psychiatric Services* 55 (2004): 886–91.

12. R. E. Drake, M. A. Wallach, and J. S. Hoffman, "Housing instability and homelessness among aftercare patients of an urban state hospital," *Hospital and Community Psychiatry* 40 (1989): 46–51; C. L. M. Caton, P. E. Shrout, P. F. Eagle, et al., "Risk factors for homelessness among schizophrenic men: A case-control study," *American Journal of Public Health* 84 (1994): 265–70; C. L. M. Caton, P. E. Shrout, B. Dominguez, et al., "Risk factors for homelessness among women with schizophrenia," ibid., 85 (1995): 1153–56; B. H. McFarland, L. R. Faulkner, J. D. Bloom, et al., "Chronic mental illness and the criminal justice system," *Hospital and Community Psychiatry* 40 (1989): 718–23; J. R. Belcher, "Are jails replacing the mental health system for the homeless mentally ill?" *Community Mental Health* 24 (1988): 185.

13. J. Bartels, R. E. Drake, M. A. Wallach, et al., "Characteristic hostility in schizophrenic outpatients," *Schizophrenia Bulletin* 17 (1991): 163–71; H. Ascher-Svanum, D. E. Faries, B. Zhu, et al., "Medication adherence and long-term functional outcomes in the treatment of schizophrenia in usual care," *Journal of Clinical Psychiatry* 67 (2006): 453–60.

14. S. Bjorkly, "Empirical evidence of a relationship between insight and risk of violence in the mentally ill—A review of the literature," *Aggression and Violent Behavior* 11 (2006): 414–23; P. F. Buckley, D. R. Hrouda, L. Friedman, et al., "Insight and its relationship to violent behavior in patients with schizophrenia," *American Journal of Psychiatry* 161 (2004): 1712–14; N. Alia-Klein, T. M. O'Rourke, R. Z. Goldstein, et al., "Insight into illness and adherence to psychotropic medications are separately associated with violence severity in a forensic sample," *Aggressive Behavior* 33 (2007): 86–96; C. Goodman, G. Knoll, V. Isakov, et al., "Insight into illness in schizophrenia," *Comprehensive Psychiatry* 46 (2005): 284–90; S. Strand, H. Belfrage, G. Fransson, et al., "Clinical and risk management factors in risk prediction of mentally disordered offenders—More important than historical data?" *Legal and Criminological Psychology* 4 (1999): 67–76; P. Woods, V. Reed, and M. Collins, "The relationship between risk and insight in a high-security forensic setting," *Journal of Psychiatric and Mental Health Nursing* 10 (2003): 510–17; M. Grevatt, B. Thomas-Peter, and G. Hughes, "Violence, mental disorder and risk assessment: Can structured clinical assessments predict the short-term risk of inpatient violence?" *Journal of Forensic Psychiatry and Psychology* 15 (2004): 278–92; S. R. Foley, B. D. Kelly, M. Clarke, et al., "Incidence and clinical correlates of aggression and violence at presentation in patients with first episode psychosis," *Schizophrenia Research* 72 (2005): 161–68; C. Arango, A. Calcedo Barba, T. González-Salvador, et al., "Violence in inpatients with schizophrenia: A prospective study," *Schizophrenia Bulletin* 25 (1999): 493–503.

15. Lanterman, "New Mental Health Legislation," speech given in Riverside, Calif., March 23, 1968.

16. Testimony of Kenneth Springer before the California Senate Select Committee on Proposed Phaseout of State Hospital Services, San Francisco, October 9, 1973.

17. *Lessard v. Schmidt*, 349 F. Supp. 1078 (E. D. Wis. 1972); T. K. Zander, "Civil com-

mitment in Wisconsin: The impact of *Lessard v. Schmidt,*" *Wisconsin Law Review* 19 (1976): 503–63.

18. *Lessard v. Schmidt.*

CHAPTER 8: THE CONSEQUENCES OF UNCONSTRAINED CIVIL LIBERTIES: HOMELESS, INCARCERATED, AND VICTIMIZED

1. D. G. Langsley and J. T. Barter, "Community mental health in California," *Western Journal of Medicine* 122 (1975): 271–76; S. P. Segal, M. A. Watson, and S. M. Goldfinger, "Civil commitment in the psychiatric emergency room," *Archives of General Psychiatry* 45 (1988): 753–58; Paul S. Applebaum, *Almost a Revolution: Mental Health Law and the Limits of Change* (New York: Oxford University Press, 1994), p. 28.

2. B. Brubaker, "HUD study of homeless quantifies the problem," *Washington Post,* March 1, 2007; Pete Earley, *Crazy: A Father's Search through America's Mental Health Madness* (New York: G. P. Putnam's Sons, 2006), p. 134; L. Gelberg and L. S. Linn, "Social and physical health of homeless adults previously treated for mental health problems," *Hospital and Community Psychiatry* 39 (1988): 510–16.

3. "Madison's top rating may attract homeless," *Wisconsin State Journal,* July 20, 1996; E. Nieves, "Homelessness tests San Francisco's ideals," *New York Times,* November 13, 1998; R. C. Archibold, "Problem of homelessness in Los Angeles and its environs draws renewed calls for action," ibid., January 15, 2006.

4. R. E. Drake, M. A. Wallach and J. S. Hoffman, "Housing instability and homelessness among aftercare patients of an urban state hospital," *Hospital and Community Psychiatry* 40 (1989): 46–51; J. R. Belcher, "Rights versus needs of homeless mentally ill persons," *Social Work* 33 (1988): 398–402; J. R. Belcher, "Defining the service needs of homeless mentally ill persons," *Hospital and Community Psychiatry* 39 (1988): 1203–5; M. Gladwell, "Backlash of the benevolent," *Washington Post,* January 22, 1995.

5. Drake et al., "Housing instability and homelessness"; L. A. Opler, L. White, C. L. M. Caton, et al., "Gender differences in the relationship of homelessness to symptom severity, substance abuse, and neuroleptic noncompliance in schizophrenia," *Journal of Nervous and Mental Disease* 189 (2001): 449–56.

6. E. Kuno, A. B. Rothbard, J. Avery, et al., "Homelessness among persons with serious mental illness in an enhanced community-based mental health system," *Psychiatric Services* 51 (2000): 1012–16.

7. G. Remal, "Police may arrest homeless man," *Kennebec* (Maine) *Journal,* September 28, 2005.

8. Earley, *Crazy,* p. 134; A. Carr, "The scary situation in our shelters," *Washington Post,* December 13, 1992.

9. L. Gelberg, L. S. Linn, and B. D. Leake, "Mental health, alcohol and drug use, and criminal history among homeless adults," *American Journal of Psychiatry* 145 (1988): 191–96; D. A. Martell, R. Rosner, and R. B. Harmon, "Base-rate estimates of criminal behavior by homeless mentally ill persons in New York City," *Psychiatric Services* 46 (1995): 596–601.

10. D. A. Martell and P. E. Dietz, "Mentally disordered offenders who push or attempt to push victims onto subway tracks in New York City," *Archives of General Psychiatry* 49 (1992): 472–75; M. Cooper, "Train suspect mentally ill, officials say," *New York Times*, April 30, 1999; N. Bernstein, "Frightening echo in tales of two in subway attacks," ibid., June 28, 1999.

11. L. Penrose, "Mental disease and crime: Outline of a comparative study of European statistics," *British Journal of Medical Psychology* 18 (1939): 1–15; G. B. Palermo, M. B. Smith, and F. J. Liska, "Jails versus mental hospitals: A social dilemma," *International Journal of Offender Therapy and Comparative Criminology* 35 (1991): 97; A. Simmons, "Prisons see more inmates requiring mental health care," *Gwinnett* (Ga.) *Daily Post*, July 30, 2006.

12. G. Swank and D. Winer, "Occurrence of psychiatric disorder in a county jail population," *American Journal of Psychiatry* 133 (1976): 1331–33.

13. Paula M. Ditton, *Mental Health and Treatment of Inmates and Probationers*, Bureau of Justice Statistics Special Report (Washington, D.C.: Department of Justice, 1999); Earley, *Crazy*, p. 44.

14. Donald M. Steinwachs, Judith D. Kasper, and Elizabeth A. Skinner, *Family Perspectives on Meeting the Needs for Care of Severely Mentally Ill Relatives: A National Survey* (Final Report to the National Alliance for the Mentally Ill by the Johns Hopkins University and University of Maryland Center on Organization and Financing of Care for the Severely Mentally Ill, Baltimore, Md., July 1992); Laura Lee Hall, Abigail C. Graf, Michael J. Fitzpatrick, et al., *TRIAD Report: Shattered Lives: Results of a National Survey of NAMI Members Living with Mental Illnesses and Their Families* (Arlington, Va.: NAMI, 2003).

15. W. Bromberg and C. B. Thompson, "The relation of psychosis, mental defect and personality types to crime," *Journal of Criminal Law and Criminology* 28 (1937): 70–88.

16. Simmons, "Prisons see more inmates requiring mental health care."

17. E. F. Torrey, J. Stieber, J. Ezekiel, et al., *Criminalizing the Seriously Mentally Ill* (Washington, D.C.: National Alliance for the Mentally Ill and Public Citizen Health Research Group, 1992), p. 60; C. Turner, "Ethical issues in criminal justice administration," *American Jails*, January/February 2007, pp. 49–53.

18. G. Simmons, "Inmate under suicide watch beaten to death," *Jackson Clarion-Ledger*, October 11, 1994; A. Guenther, "Family sues Camco over prisoner's death," (New Jersey) *Courier-Post*, June 14, 2006.

19. M. C. Ford, "Frequent fliers: High demand users of local corrections," *American Jails*, July/August 2005, pp. 18–26; L. Kilzer, "Jail as a 'halfway house' . . . or long-term commitment?" *Denver Post*, June 3, 1984; S. Downing, "Mentally ill woman sent to state facility," (Memphis) *Commercial Appeal*, March 10, 1999; Earley, *Crazy*, p. 79.

20. *Criminal Justice/Mental Health Consensus Project*, www.consensusproject.org, accessed July 19, 2006.

21. E. V. Valdisseri, K. R. Carroll, and A. J. Hartl, "A study of offenses committed by psychotic inmates in a county jail," *Hospital and Community Psychiatry* 37 (1986): 163–65; Torrey et al., *Criminalizing the Seriously Mentally Ill*; Early, *Crazy*; S. Had-

dock, "Mental illness training help Cache police," (Salt Lake City) *Deseret News*, October 7, 1999.

22. J. Barbanel, "10 homeless people held at Bellevue Mental Unit," *New York Times*, October 30, 1987; "The mental health sieve" (editorial), ibid., October 2, 1988; E. Bumiller, "In wake of attack, Giuliani cracks down on homeless," ibid., November 20, 1999; N. Bernstein, "Qualms about police rules on handling the mentally ill," ibid., September 1, 1999; J. Caldwell Bonovitz and J. S. Bonovitz, "Diversion of the mentally ill into the criminal justice system: The police intervention perspective," *American Journal of Psychiatry* 138 (1981): 973–76.

23. J. Strong, "Battling their demons," *Des Moines Register*, September 14, 2006.

24. "Homicide trends in the U.S.: Number of justifiable homicides" (www.ojp.usdoj.gov/bjs/homicide/tables/justifytab.htm) and "Justifiable homicides by police" (www.ojp.usdoj.gov/bjs/homicide/tables/justifyreasontab.htm) (Washington, D.C.: U.S. Department of Justice, 2006).

25. Anthony Baez Foundation, National Lawyers Guild, and October 22nd Coalition to Stop Police Brutality, Repression, and the Criminalization of a Generation, *Stolen Lives, Killed by Law Enforcement*, 2nd ed. (New York: Stolen Lives Project, 1999); J. J. Frye, "Policing the emotionally disturbed," *Journal of the American Academy of Psychiatry and the Law* 28 (2000): 345–47; "Mental illness frequently deepens tragedy of police shootings," *Seattle Post-Intelligencer*, May 25, 2000; Ventura County Grand Jury Report, *Fatal Shootings in Ventura County by Law Enforcement Officers, 1992–2001* (Office of Ventura County District Attorney).

26. "A ferocious crime against the helpless" (editorial), *Cape Cod Times*, July 22, 1984.

27. Sheila Broughel's tragedy is detailed by Rael Jean Isaac and Virginia C. Armat in *Madness in the Streets: How Psychiatry and the Law Abandoned the Mentally Ill* (New York: Free Press, 1990), pp. 260–65.

28. Phyllis Iannotta's death is detailed by B. Kates in *The Murder of a Shopping Bag Lady* (New York: Harcourt Brace Jovanovich, 1985).

29. A. F. Lehman and L. S. Linn, "Crimes against discharged mental patients in board-and-care homes," *American Journal of Psychiatry* 141 (1984): 271–74; S. Friedman and G. Harrison, "Sexual histories, attitudes, and behavior of schizophrenic and 'normal' women," *Archives of Sexual Behavior* 13 (1984): 555–67.

30. "Face now has a name, but slaying baffles Va. authorities," *Washington Post*, July 13, 1988; M. Lembede, "Man charged in homeless woman's death," ibid., August 30, 1988; L. A. Goodman, M. A. Dutton, and M. Harris, "Episodically homeless women with serious mental illness: Prevalence of physical and sexual assault," *American Journal of Orthopsychiatry* 65 (1995): 468–78.

31. T. Alex, "Summer in the city: Violent crime in D.M.," *Des Moines Register*, August 3, 1989; D. Lorch, "Death of a homeless man: From ivy league to streets," *New York Times*, November 20, 1990; Nieves, "Homelessness tests San Francisco's ideals."

32. E. Silver, "Mental disorder and violent victimization: The mediating role of involvement in conflicted social relationships," *Criminology* 40 (2002): 191–212; J. S. Brekke, C. Prindle, S. W. Bae, et al., "Risks for individuals with schizophrenia who are living in the community," *Psychiatric Services* 52 (2001): 1358–66.

33. Brekke et al., "Risk for individuals with schizophrenia"; J. S. Gearon, A. S. Bel-

lack, and C. H. Brown, "Sexual and physical abuse in women with schizophrenia: Prevalence and risk factors" (abstract), *Schizophrenia Research* 60 (2003): 38; V. A. Hiday, M. S. Swartz, J. W. Swanson, et al., "Impact of outpatient commitment on victimization of people with severe mental illness," *American Journal of Psychiatry* 159 (2002): 1403-11.

34. L. A. Teplin, G. M. McClelland, K. M. Abram, et al., "Crime victimization in adults with severe mental illness," *Archives of General Psychiatry* 62 (2005): 911-21.

35. C. J. Levy, "Voiceless, defenseless and a source of cash," *New York Times*, April 30, 2002; C. J. Levy, "Doctor admits he did needless surgery on the mentally ill," ibid., May 20, 2003; C. J. Levy, "Home for mentally ill settles suit on coerced prostate surgery for $7.4 million," ibid., August 5, 2004; "Group-home owners charged with resident abuse, fraud," *Washington Post*, November 8, 2005.

CHAPTER 9: THE CONSEQUENCES OF UNCONSTRAINED CIVIL LIBERTIES: VIOLENT AND HOMICIDAL

1. M. S. Swartz, J. W. Swanson, V. A. Hiday, et al., "Violence and severe mental illness: The effects of substance abuse and nonadherence to medication," *American Journal of Psychiatry* 155 (1998): 226-31.

2. Donald M. Steinwachs, Judith D. Kasper, and Elizabeth A. Skinner, *Family Perspectives on Meeting the Needs for Care of Severely Mentally Ill Relatives: A National Survey* (Final Report to the National Alliance for the Mentally Ill by the Johns Hopkins University and University of Maryland Center on Organization and Financing of Care for the Severely Mentally Ill, Baltimore, Md., July 1992).

3. J. W. Swanson, M. S. Swartz, R. A. Van Dorn, et al., "A national study of violent behavior in persons with schizophrenia," *Archives of General Psychiary* 63 (2006): 490-99.

4. H. J. Steadman, E. P. Mulvey, J. Monahan, et al., "Violence by people discharged from acute psychiatric inpatient facilities and by others in the same neighborhoods," *Archives of General Psychiatry* 55 (1998): 393-401; H. J. Steadman and E. Silver, "Immediate precursors of violence among persons with mental illness: A return to a situational perspective," in *Violence among the Mentally Ill* (Boston: Kluwer Academic Publishers, 1999), pp. 35-48.

5. See note 3 above.

6. J. Monahan, H. J. Steadman, P. C. Robbins, et al., "An actuarial model of violence risk assessment for persons with mental disorders," *Psychiatric Services* 56 (2005): 810-15.

7. J. W. Swanson, C. E. Holzer, V. K. Ganju, et al., "Violence and psychiatric disorder in the community: Evidence from the Epidemiologic Catchment Area Surveys," *Hospital and Community Psychiatry* 41 (1990): 761-70; J. W. Swanson, "Mental disorder, substance abuse, and community violence: An epidemiological approach," in J. Monahan and H. J. Steadman, *Violence and Mental Disorder: Developments in Risk Assessment* (Chicago: University of Chicago Press, 1994), pp. 101-36.

8. J. Milton, S. Amin, S. P. Singh, et al., "Aggressive incidents in first-episode psychosis," *British Journal of Psychiatry* 178 (2001): 433-48; M. Doyle and M. Dolan, "Predicting community violence from patients discharged from mental health

services," ibid., 189 (2006): 520–26; E. Walsh, C. Gilvarry, C. Samele, et al., "Predicting violence in schizophrenia: A prospective study," *Schizophrenia Research* 67 (2004): 247–52.

9. S. Hodgins, "Mental disorder, intellectual deficiency, and crime," *Archives of General Psychiatry* 49 (1992): 476–83.

10. J. Tiihonen, M. Isohanni, P. Räsänen, et al., "Specific major mental disorders and criminality: A 26-year prospective study of the 1966 Northern Finland Birth Cohort," *American Journal of Psychiatry* 154 (1997): 840–45; S. Hodgins, S. A. Mednick, P. A. Brennan, et al., "Mental disorder and crime," *Archives of General Psychiatry* 53 (1996): 489–96; P. A. Brennan, S. A. Mednick, and S. Hodgins, "Major mental disorders and criminal violence in a Danish Birth Cohort," ibid., 57 (2000): 494–500; L. Arseneault, T. E. Moffitt, A. Caspi, et al., "Mental disorders and violence in a total birth cohort," ibid., 979–86.

11. F. Grunberg, B. I. Klinger, and B. Grumet, "Homicide and deinstitutionalization of the mentally ill," *American Journal of Psychiatry* 134 (1977): 685–87; F. Grunberg, B. I. Klinger, and B. R. Grumet, "Homicide and community-based psychiatry," *Journal of Nervous and Mental Disease* 166 (1978): 868–74.

12. D. E. Wilcox, "The relationship of mental illness to homicide," *American Journal of Forensic Psychiatry* 6 (1985): 3–15.

13. John M. Dawson and Patrick A. Langan, *Murder in Families* (Washington, D.C.: Bureau of Justice Statistics, U.S. Department of Justice, 1994).

14. H. Pétursson and G. H. Gudjónsson, "Psychiatric aspects of homicide," *Acta Psychiatrica Scandinavica* 64 (1981): 363–72.

15. F. Fessenden, "Rampage killers: They threaten, seethe and unhinge, then kill in quantity," *New York Times*, April 9, 2000, p. 1; L. Goldstein and W. Glaberson, "Rampage killers: The well-marked roads to homicidal rage," ibid., April 10, 2000.

16. Personal communication, FBI data from Ford Fessenden, May 2, 2000.

17. A. G. Hempel, J. R. Meloy, and T. C. Richards, "Offender and offense characteristics of a nonrandom sample of mass murderers," *Journal of the American Academy of Psychiatry and the Law* 27 (1999): 213–25.

18. D. B. Roddy and M. Rosenwald, "Taylor kept a 'Satan List,' " *Pittsburgh Post-Gazette*, March 3, 2000; T. Spangler, "Five slain in Pennsylvania shootings," *Washington Post*, April 29, 2000.

19. M. E. Ruane, "Looking back . . . we should have done something," *Washington Post*, April 22, 2007; M. E. Ruane and C. L. Jenkins, "Gunman sent video during lull in slaughter," ibid., April 19, 2007; N. R. Kleinfield, "Before deadly rage, a lifetime consumed by a troubling silence," *New York Times*, April 22, 2007; M. Shuchman, "Falling through the cracks—Virginia Tech and the restructuring of college mental health services," *New England Journal of Medicine* 357 (2007): 105–10.

20. Dawson and Langan, *Murder in Families*.

21. C. C. Joyal, A. Putkonen, P. Paavola, et al., "Characteristics and circumstances of homicidal acts committed by offenders with schizophrenia," *Psychological Medicine* 34 (2004): 433–42; K. A. Straznickas, D. E. McNiel, and R. L. Binder, "Violence toward family caretakers by mentally ill relatives," *Hospital and Community Psychiatry* 44 (1993): 385–87.

22. R. Martindale, "Couple lives in fear of schizophrenic son's return," *Tulsa World,* June 24, 1984; C. Acker, "Families under siege: A mental health crisis," *Philadelphia Inquirer,* September 10, 1989; J. Doe, "My brother might kill me," *New York Times,* May 6, 1987; Ellen L., "The other terrorism," *NAMI Maryland* newsletter, Winter 2002, p. 5.

23. C. Acker and M. J. Fine, "Using the threat of jail as protection," *Philadelphia Inquirer,* September 14, 1989.

24. Nona Dearth, B. J. Labenski, M. E. Mott, et al., *Families Helping Families: Living with Schizophrenia* (New York: W. W. Norton, 1986).

25. A. Nordström and G. Kullgren, "Victim relations and victim gender in violent crimes committed by offenders with schizophrenia," *Social Psychiatry and Psychiatric Epidemiology* 38 (2003): 326–30; C. M. Green, "Matricide by sons," *Medicine, Science and the Law* 21 (1981): 207–14; S. Wessely, "Psychopathology of violence (letter)," *Lancet* 2 (1987): 801; A. Nordström and G. Kullgren, "Do violent offenders with schizophrenia who attack family members differ from those with other victims?" *International Journal of Forensic Mental Health* 2 (2003): 195–200.

26. E. Lichtblau and T. Drummond, "Did mental care system fail Betty Madeira," *Los Angeles Times,* October 21, 1990, pp. B1, B5; T. Jackman, "Va. man who killed mother to be freed," *Washington Post,* July 9, 2005; D. Hench, "Troubled son held in mom's slaying," *Portland Press-Herald,* June 22, 2006.

27. A. M. Weisman and K. K. Sharma, "Forensic analysis and psycholegal implications of parricide and attempted parricide," *Journal of Forensic Sciences* 42 (1997): 1107–13; B. Rankin, "Another senseless tragic odyssey," *The* (California AMI) *Journal,* Fall 1990, pp. 11–13; Associated Press, "Mentally ill man kills father, eats brain," March 23, 1997.

28. J. Simerman and K. Fischer, "Again, a son arrested in parent's killing," *Contra Costa Times,* February 22, 2007.

29. P. J. Resnick, "Child murder by parents: A psychiatric review of filicide," *American Journal of Psychiatry* 126 (1969): 325–34; S. H. Friedman, S. M. Horwitz and P. J. Resnick, "Child murder by mothers: A critical analysis of the current state of knowledge and a research agenda," *American Journal of Psychiatry* 162 (2005): 1578–87; "Swedish parents kill 258 of their children (1965–1999)," press release for the Society for Promotion of Community Standards Inc., July 28, 2006, http://www.scoop.co.nz/stories/PO0607/S00364.htm, accessed August 3, 2006.

30. Associated Press, "Yates sentenced to life as family debates blame," *Washington Post,* March 19, 2002, p. A6.

31. S. Hatters Friedman, D. R. Hrouda, C. E. Holden, et al., "Child murder committed by severely mentally ill mothers: An examination of mothers found not guilty by reason of insanity," *Journal of Forensic Sciences* 50 (2005): 1466–71.

32. F. Bruni, "Behind jokes, a life of pain and delusion," *New York Times,* November 22, 1998.

33. P. E. Mullen, M. Pathé, R. Purcell, et al., "Study of stalkers," *American Journal of Psychiatry* 156 (1999): 1244–49.

34. E. Fuller Torrey, Peter Lurie, Sidney M. Wolfe, et al., *Threats to Radio and Television Station Personnel in the United States by Individuals with Severe Mental Illnesses* (Wash-

ington, D.C. Public Citizen's Health Research Group and Treatment Advocacy Center, 1999).

35. R. Morell, "Suspect left mixed impressions," *Charlotte Observer*, September 2, 1994.

36. H. S. Moran, "KSL suspect delusional, attorney says," (Salt Lake City) *Deseret News*, January 29, 1999.

37. D. Shore, C. R. Filson, and D. S. Rae, "Violent crime arrest rates of White House Case subjects and matched control subjects," *American Journal of Psychiatry* 147 (1990): 746–50.

38. F. Butterfield, "Killing of 2 nuns prompts questioning of mental care," *New York Times*, January 31, 1996.

39. "Devils, delusions, murder," *Hartford Courant*, August 25, 2002.

40. B. Lambert, "Man guilty of killing priest and parishioner," *New York Times*, June 26, 2003.

41. R. A. Friedman, "Violence and mental illness—How strong is the link?" *New England Journal of Medicine* 355 (2006): 2064–66; K. M. Song, "Mental-health work can be fatal," *Seattle Times*, September 15, 2006.

42. J. D. Bloom, "The character of danger in psychiatric practice: Are the mentally ill dangerous?" *Bulletin of the American Academy of Psychiatry and the Law* 17 (1989): 241–55.

43. J. Wilson, "Cops: Cyanide plotter had hit lists," Associated Press, August 25, 1998.

44. Bloom, "The character of danger: Killer called 'very, very sick,' " *Washington Post*, June 13, 1999; S. Siegel, "Man pleads guilty to murdering psychiatrist," (Montgomery County, Md.) *Gazette*, April 4, 2007.

45. D. D. Lacy, "Psychiatric nurse attacked and killed on the job," *The* (New York State Public Employees Federation) *Communicator*, February 1999; Song, "Mental-health work can be fatal."

46. M. Eronen, P. Hakola, and J. Tiihonen, "Factors associated with homicide recidivism in a 13-year sample of homicide offenders in Finland," *Psychiatric Services* 47 (1996): 403–6.

47. H. R. Lamb, "Incompetency to stand trial," *Archives of General Psychiatry* 44 (1987): 754–58.

48. B. Miller, "Woman freed on insanity plea held in new slaying," *Washington Post*, July 10, 1993; P. Davis and B. Miller, "Police had warning of violence," ibid., July 13, 1993; S. Twomey, "When insanity collides with humanity," ibid., July 15, 1993; S. James, "After '75 murders of his family, Detroit man again accused of killing family," *Detroit Free Press*, January 28, 2000; Associated Press, "Need seen to plug holes in care of mentally ill," February 21, 1999.

49. L. Hicks, "Insanity ruling frees him—again," *Des Moines Register*, June 26, 1999.

CHAPER 10: AN IMPERATIVE FOR CHANGE

1. J. Swanson, R. Borum, M. Swartz, et al., "Violent behavior preceding hospitalization among persons with severe mental illness," *Law and Human Behavior* 23 (1999): 185–204.

2. S. Rachlin, A. Pam, and J. Milton, "Civil liberties versus involuntary hospitalization," *American Journal of Psychiatry* 132 (1975): 189–92.

3. D. Treffert, "Legal 'rites': Criminalizing the mentally ill," *Hillside Journal of Clinical Psychiatry* 3 (1982): 122–37.

4. John Locke, *Two Treatises of Government* (1690), in Peter Laslett, ed., *Two Treatises of Government: A Critical Edition* (London: Mentor, 1967), pp. 348–52.

5. Otto F. Wahl, *Telling Is Risky Business: Mental Health Consumers Confront Stigma* (New Brunswick: Rutgers University Press, 1999), p. 15.

6. J. C. Phelan, B. G. Link, A. Stueve, et al., "Public conceptions of mental illness in 1950 and 1996: What is mental illness and is it to be feared?" *Journal of Health and Social Behavior* 41 (2000): 188–207.

7. B. G. Link, F. T. Cullen, J. Frank, et al., "The social rejection of former mental patients: Understanding why labels matter," *American Journal of Sociology* 92 (1987): 1461–1500.

8. H. R. Lamb, "Combating stigma by providing treatment," *Psychiatric Services* 50 (1999): 729.

9. H. A. Phelps, "Rhode Island's threat against murder," *Journal of Criminal Law and Criminology* 15 (1925): 552–67; L. I. Dublin and B. Bunzel, "Thou shalt not kill: A study of homicide in the United States," *Survey Graphic* 24 (1935): 127–39; J. H. Cassity, "Personality study of 200 murderers," *Journal of Criminal Psychopathology* 2 (1941): 296–304; Marvin E. Wolfgang, *Patterns in Criminal Homicide* (New York: John Wiley, 1966, originally published in 1958), p. 314; a fifth study of homicides in Detroit is not comparable, since it included sexual crimes under the category of mentally ill (J. Boudouris, "A classification of homicides," *Criminology* 11 (1974): 525–40.

10. F. Grunberg, B. I. Klinger, and B. Grumet, "Homicide and deinstitutionalization of the mentally ill," *American Journal of Psychiatry* 134 (1977): 685–87; K. Tardiff, P. M. Marzuk, A. C. Leon, et al., "Violence by patients admitted to a private psychiatric hospital," ibid., 154 (1997): 88–93; D. A. Martell and P. E. Dietz, "Mentally disordered offenders who push or attempt to push victims onto subway tracks in New York City," *Archives of General Psychiatry* 49 (1992): 472–75; Ford Fessenden, personal communication, May 2, 2000; J. Heller, "Potential violence looms when they share a home," *San Diego Union-Tribune*, August 13, 2001.

11. "Health care reform for Americans with severe mental illnesses: Report of the National Advisory Mental Health Council," *American Journal of Psychiatry* 150 (1993): 1447–65; H. Harwood, A. Ameen, G. Denmead, et al., *The Economic Cost of Mental Illness* (Rockville, Md.: National Institute of Mental Health, NIH, July 2000), pp. 1–2.

12. L. M. Davies and M. F. Drummond, "Economics and schizophrenia: The real cost," *British Journal of Psychiatry* 165, suppl. 25 (1994): 18–21.

13. T. L. Mark, R. M. Coffey, E. King, et al., "Spending on mental health and substance abuse treatment, 1987–1997," *Health Affairs* 19 (2000): 108–20; SSI and SSDI data are taken from the Social Security Administration's *Annual Statistical Supplements to the Social Security Bulletin* (Washington, D.C.: Government Printing Office, 1987, 1998, 2002).

14. T. W. Haywood, H. M. Kravitz, L. S. Grossman, et al., "Predicting the 'Revolving Door' " phenomenon among patients with schizophrenic, schizoaffective, and affective disorders," *American Journal of Psychiatry* 152 (1995): 856–61.

15. R. Davidson, "A mental health crisis in Illinois," *Chicago Tribune*, December 9, 1991; B. Herbert, "Mental health failures," *New York Times*, September 5, 1993; J. L. Geller, "A report on the 'worst' state hospital recidivists in the U.S.," *Hospital and Community Psychiatry* 43 (1992): 904–8; Annette McGaha and Paul Stiles, *Florida Mental Health Act (Baker Act) 2001 Annual Report* (Tampa, Fla.: Louis de la Parte Florida Mental Health Institute, 2002).

16. M. Gladwell, "A brush with madness," *Washington Post*, May 12, 1993.

17. D. F. Eslinger, "Personal tragedy far from only catalyst," *Catalyst* (newsletter of the Treatment Advocacy Center), Summer 2004; I. Goldstrom, M. Henderson, A. Male, et al., "Jail mental health services: A national survey," in R. W. Manderscheid and M. J. Henderson, eds., *Mental Health, United States, 1998*, DHHS Publication No. (SMA) 99–3285 (Washington, D.C.: U.S. Department of Health and Human Services, Substance Abuse and Mental Health Services Administration, Center for Mental Health Services, 1998), pp. 176–87; L. T. Izumi, M. Schiller, and S. Hayward, *Corrections, Criminal Justice, and the Mentally Ill: Some Observations about Costs in California* (San Francisco: Pacific Research Institute for Public Policy, 1996).

18. "Jailed schizophrenic awarded $5.4 M," *AP Online*, March 11, 1999; T. Jackman, "Reston family sues in insanity case," *Washington Post*, October 1, 2000; news story, WREG, Memphis, Tenn., May 21, 2004; A. Guenther, "Family sues Camco over prisoner's death," (New Jersey) *Courier Post*, June 14, 2006; P. Belluck, "Mentally ill inmates at risk in isolation, lawsuit says," *New York Times*, March 9, 2007.

19. J. Monahan and H. J. Steadman, "Crime and mental disorder: An epidemiological approach," in Michael Tonry and Norval Morris, eds., *Crime and Justice: A Criminological Review of Research* (Chicago: University of Chicago Press, 1983), 181–82.

20. J. Monahan, "Mental disorder and violent behavior," *American Psychologist* 47 (1992): 511–21.

21. H. J. Steadman, E. P. Mulvey, J. Monahan, et al., "Violence by people discharged from acute psychiatric inpatient facilities and by others in the same neighborhoods," *Archives of General Psychiatry* 55 (1998): 393–401; "Discharged mental patients without substance abuse exhibit same rate of violence as non-mentally ill neighbors, study finds," press release of the University of Virginia School of Law, May 14, 1998; "Violence study dispels perception of psychiatric patients," *Mental Health Weekly* 8 (1998): 1, 4; S. G. Boodman, "Are former mental patients more violent?" *Washington Post*, May 19, 1998.

22. F. Butterfield, "Studies of mental illness show links to violence," *New York Times*, May 15, 1998.

23. H. J. Steadman and E. Silver, "Immediate precursors of violence among persons with mental illness: A return to a situational perspective," in S. Hodgins, ed., *Violence among the Mentally Ill* (Boston: Kluwer Academic Publishers, 1999), pp. 35–48.

24. G. Cote, "Commentary," in Hodgins, ed., *Violence among the Mentally Ill*, p. 52.

25. John Monahan, Henry J. Steadman, Eric Silver, et al., *Rethinking Risk Assessment: The MacArthur Study of Mental Disorder and Violence* (Oxford: Oxford University Press, 2001), p. 137.

26. J. Campbell, S. Stefan, and A. Loder, "Putting violence in context," *Hospital and Community Psychiatry* 45 (1994): 633.

27. P. J. Taylor and J. Gunn, "Homicides by people with mental illness: Myth and reality," *British Journal of Psychiatry* 174 (1999): 9–14.

28. Hearings on the Select Committee on Proposed Phaseout of State Hospital Services, May 18 to October 10, 1973, California State Archives, and quoted in J. Chase, "Where have all the patients gone?" *Human Behavior* 2 (1973): 14–21.

29. F. Grunberg, B. I. Klinger, and B. B. Grumet, "Homicide and community-based psychiatry," *Journal of Nervous and Mental Disease* 166 (1978): 868–74.

30. D. E. Wilcox, "The relationship of mental illness to homicide," *American Journal of Forensic Psychiatry* 6 (1985): 3–10.

31. P. Noble, "Crime, violence and schizophrenia" (letter), *British Journal of Psychiatry* 171 (1997): 189–90; J. W. Swanson and C. E. Holzer III, "Violence and ECA data (letter)," *Hospital and Community Psychiatry* 42 (1991): 954–55; P. E. Mullen, "Schizophrenia and violence: From correlations to preventive strategies," *Advances in Psychiatric Treatment* 12 (2006): 239–48.

CHAPTER 11: FIXING THE SYSTEM

1. M. B. Pfeiffer, "Let's care for the weakest among us," *Miami Herald*, November 29, 2006.

2. B. McKelway, "Va. chief justice leads the start of effort to revise state's laws," *Richmond Times-Dispatch*, September 2, 2006; H. Ascher-Svanum, D. E. Faries, B. Zhu, et al., "Medication adherence and long-term functional outcomes in the treatment of schizophrenia in usual care," *Journal of Clinical Psychiatry* 67 (2006): 453–60; W. H. Fisher and K. M. Roy-Bujnowski, "Patterns and prevalence of arrest in a statewide cohort of mental health care consumers," *Psychiatric Services* 57 (2006): 1623–28.

3. L. M. Davies and M. F. Drummond, "Economics and schizophrenia: The real cost," *British Journal of Psychiatry* 165, suppl. 25 (1994): 18–21.

4. P. Räsänen, J. Tiihonen, M. Isohanni, et al., *Schizophrenia Bulletin* 24 (1998): 437–41; C. Wallace, P. Mullen, P. Burgess, et al., "Serious criminal offending and mental disorder," *British Journal of Psychiatry* 172 (1998): 477–84.

5. N. Alia-Klein, T. M. O'Rourke, R. Z. Goldstein, et al., "Insight into illness and adherence to psychotropic medications are separately associated with violence severity in a forensic sample," *Aggressive Behavior* 33 (2007): 86–96; P. F. Buckley, D. R. Hrouda, L. Friedman, et al., "Insight and its relationship to violent behavior in patients with schizophrenia," *American Journal of Psychiatry* 161 (2004): 1712–14; D. Hrouda, P. J. Resnick, L. Friedman, et al., "Violence and schizophrenia: Further observations on standards of care" (abstract), *Schizophrenia Research* 60 (2003): 40; S. J. Bertels, R. E. Drake, M. A. Wallach, et al., "Characteristic hostility in schizophrenic outpatients," *Schizophrenia Bulletin* 17 (1991): 163–71; H. Ascher-Svanum,

D. E. Faries, B. Zhu, et al., "Medication adherence and long-term functional outcomes in the treatment of schizophrenia in usual care," *Journal of Clinical Psychiatry* 67 (2006): 453–60. See also S. Strand, H. Belfrage, G. Fransson, et al., "Clinical and risk management factors in risk prediction of mentally disordered offenders— More important than historical data?" *Legal and Criminological Psychology* 4 (1999): 67–76; P. Woods, V. Reed, and M. Collins, "The relationship between risk and insight in a high-security forensic setting," *Journal of Psychiatric and Mental Health Nursing* 10 (2003): 510–17; M. Grevatt, B. Thomas-Peter, and G. Hughes, "Violence, mental disorder and risk assessment: Can structured clinical assessments predict the short-term risk of inpatient violence?" *Journal of Forensic Psychiatry and Psychology* 15 (2004): 278–92; S. R. Foley, B. D. Kelly, M. Clarke, et al., "Incidence and clinical correlates of aggression and violence at presentation in patients with first episode psychosis," *Schizophrenia Research* 72 (2005): 161–68; M. S. Swartz, J. W. Swanson, V. A. Hiday, et al., "Violence and severe mental illness: The effects of substance abuse and nonadherence to medication," *American Journal of Psychiatry* 155 (1998): 226–31; L. D. Smith, "Medication refusal and the rehospitalized mentally ill inmate," *Hospital and Community Psychiatry* 40 (1989): 491–96; J. A. Yesavage, "Inpatient violence and the schizophrenic patient: An inverse correlation between danger-related events and neuroleptic levels," *Biological Psychiatry* 17 (1982): 1331–37; K. E. Weaver, "Increasing the dose of antipsychotic medication to control violence," (letter) *American Journal of Psychiatry* 140 (1983): 1274; J. A. Kasper, S. K. Hoge, T. Feucht-Haviar, et al., "Prospective study of patients' refusal of antipsychotic medication under a physician discretion review procedure," *American Journal of Psychiatry* 154 (1997): 483–89; T. Steinert, T. Sippach, and R. P. Gebhardt, "How common is violence in schizophrenia despite neuroleptic treatment?" *Pharmacopsychiatry* 33 (2000): 98–102.

6. A. Tengström, S. Hodgins, and G. Kullgren, "Men with schizophrenia who behave violently: The usefulness of an early- versus late-start offender typology," *Schizophrenia Bulletin* 27 (2001): 205–18. See also K. A. Nolan, J. Volavka, P. Mohr, et al., "Psychopathy and violent behavior among patients with schizophrenia or schizoaffective disorder," *Psychiatric Services* 50 (1999): 787–92.

7. S. Bjørkly, "Psychotic symptoms and violence toward others—A literature review of some preliminary findings: Part 1. Delusions," *Aggression and Violent Behavior* 7 (2002): 617–31; B. G. Link, J. Monahan, A. Stueve, et al., "Real in their consequences: A sociological approach to understanding the association between psychotic symptoms and violence," *American Sociological Review* 64 (1999): 316–32; K. Hersh and R. Borum, "Command hallucinations, compliance, and risk assessment," *Journal of the American Academy of Psychiatry and the Law* 26 (1998): 353–59.

8. M. Krakowski, P. Czobor, and J. C.-Y. Chou, "Course of violence in patients with schizophrenia: Relationship to clinical symptoms," *Schizophrenia Bulletin* 25 (1999): 505–17; K. Naudts and S. Hodgins, "Neurological correlates of violent behavior among persons with schizophrenia," ibid., 32 (2006): 562–72; M. Das, V. Kumari, I. Barkataki, et al., "Anticipatory fear in violent schizophrenia and personality disorder subjects: A functional MRI study (abstract)," *Biological Psychiatry* 55 (2004): 70S.

9. M. Krakowski and P. Czobor, "Gender differences in violent behaviors: Relationship to clinical symptoms and psychosocial factors," *American Journal of Psychiatry* 161 (2004): 459–65; J. N. Lam, D. E. McNiel, and R. L. Binder, "The relationship between patients' gender and violence leading to staff injuries," *Psychiatric Services* 51 (2000): 1167–70; H. Schanda, G. Knecht, D. Schreinzer, et al., "Homicide and major mental disorders: A 25-year study," *Acta Psychiatrica Scandinavica* 110 (2004): 98–107; A. I. F. Simpson, B. McKenna, A. Moskowitz, et al., "Homicide and mental illness in New Zealand, 1970–2000," *British Journal of Psychiatry* 185 (2004): 394–98.

10. Swartz, et al., "Violence and severe mental illness."

11. J. Monahan and H. J. Steadman, eds., *Violence and Mental Disorder: Developments in Risk Assessment* (Chicago: University of Chicago Press, 1994); J. Monahan, H. J. Steadman, E. Silver, et al., *Rethinking Risk Assessment: The MacArthur Study of Mental Disorder and Violence* (New York: Oxford University Press, 2001); J. Monahan and H. J. Steadman, "Violent storms and violent people: How meteorology can inform risk communication in mental health law," *American Psychologist* 51 (1996): 931–38; C. L. Scott and P. J. Resnick, "Violence risk assessment in persons with mental illness," *Aggression and Violent Behavior* 11 (2006): 598–611.

12. M. Tran, K. Pang, and H. G. Reza, "Sniper's family recalls him as a 'sweetheart': His mother and son say Henry Lee Brown was a caring man when he took his schizophrenia medication," *Los Angeles Times*, June 16, 2004.

13. D. J. Allness and W. H. Knoedler, *The PACT Model of Community-Based Treatment for Persons with Severe and Persistent Mental Illness* (Arlington, Va.: NAMI, 1998).

14. Mary Flannery and Mark Glickman, *Fountain House: Portraits of Lives Reclaimed from Mental Illness* (Center City, Minn.: Hazelden, 1996).

15. Steinert et al., "How common is violence in schizophrenia"; L. F. Dailey, S. W. Townsend, M. W. Dysken, et al., "Recidivism in medication-noncompliant serious juvenile offenders with bipolar disorder," *Journal of Clinical Psychiatry* 66 (2005): 477–84.

16. L. Citrome, J. Valavka, P. Czobor, et al., "Effects of clozapine, olanzapine, risperidone, and haloperidol on hostility among patients with schizophrenia," *Psychiatric Services* 52 (2001): 1510–14; M. I. Krakowski, P. Czobor, L. Citrome, et al., "Atypical antipsychotic agents in the treatment of violent patients with schizophrenia and schizoaffective disorder," *Archives of General Psychiatry* 63 (2006): 622–29; J. Volavka, "Treatment approaches to aggressive behavior in schizophrenia," in Adrian Raine, ed., *Crime and Schizophrenia: Causes and Cures* (Hauppauge, N.Y.: Nova Science Publishers, 2006), pp. 301–14; W. G. Frankel, D. Shera, H. Berger-Hershkowitz, et al., "Clozapine-associated reduction in arrest rates of psychotic patients with criminal histories," *American Journal of Psychiatry* 158 (2001): 270–74; L. Citrome, "The psychopharmacology of violence with emphasis on schizophrenia: Part 2. Long-term treatment," *Journal of Clinical Psychiatry* 68 (2007): 331–32.

17. P. Jorgensen, "Recovery and insight in schizophrenia," *Acta Psychiatrica Scandinavica* 92 (1995): 436–40; M. A. Weiler, M. H. Fleisher, and D. McArthur-Campbell, "Insight and symptom change in schizophrenia and other disorders," *Schizophre-*

nia Research 45 (2000): 29–36; C. Henry and S. N. Ghaemi, "Insight in psychosis: A systematic review of treatment interventions," *Psychopathology* 37 (2004): 194–99; G. M. Gharabawi, R. A. Lasser, C. A. Bossie, et al., "Insight and its relationship to clinical outcomes in patients with schizophrenia or schizoaffective disorder receiving long-acting risperidone," *International Clinical Psychopharmacology* 21 (2006): 233–40.

18. M. Sherrill, "Out There: They are homeless, hopeless, wretched, heartbreaking, cunning, grungy, needy, greedy, idle, hungry, angry, aggravating. And ours," *Washington Post*, January 19, 1992; B. A. Pescosolido, J. Monahan, B. G. Link, et al., "The public's view of the competence, dangerousness, and need for legal coercion of persons with mental health problems," *American Journal of Public Health* 89 (1999): 1339–45.

19. D. J. Luchins, P. Hanrahan, K. J. Conrad, et al, "An agency-based representative payee program and improved community tenure of persons with mental illness," *Psychiatric Services* 49 (1998): 1218–22; K. J. Conrad, G. Lutz, M. D. Matters, et al., "Randomized trial of psychiatric care with representative payeeship for persons with serious mental illness," ibid., 57 (2006): 197–204; P. S. Applebaum and A. Redlich, "Use of leverage over patients' money to promote adherence to psychiatric treatment," *Journal of Nervous and Mental Disease* 194 (2006): 294–302.

20. P. C. Robbins, J. Petrila, S. LeMelle, et al., "The use of housing as leverage to increase adherence to psychiatric treatment in the community," *Administration and Policy in Mental Health and Mental Health Services Research* 33 (2006); 226–36.

21. A. D. Redlich, H. J. Steadman, J. Monahan, et al., "Patterns of practice in mental health courts: A national survey," *Law and Human Behavior* 30 (2006): 347–62; H. Herinckx, S. Swart, S. Ama, et al., *The Clark County Mentally Ill Re-Arrest Prevention (MIRAP) Program, Final Evaluation Report* (Portland, Ore.: Regional Research Institute for Human Services, Portland State University, 2003); M. S. Ridgely, J. Engberg, M. D. Greenberg, et al., "Justice, treatment, and cost—An evaluation of the fiscal impact of Allegheny County Mental Health Court," RAND Technical Report, available at www.rand.org/pubs/technical_reports/TR439, accessed August 2, 2007.

22. C. O'Keefe, D. P. Potenza, and K. T. Mueser, "Treatment outcomes for severely mentally ill patients on conditional discharge to community-based treatment," *Journal of Nervous and Mental Disease* 185 (1997): 409–11.

23. D. A. Bigelow, J. D. Bloom, and M. H. Williams, "Costs of managing insanity acquittees under a Psychiatric Security Review Board system," *Hospital and Community Psychiatry* 41 (1990): 613–14; Joseph D. Bloom and Mary H. Williams, *Management and Treatment of Insanity Acquittees: A Model for the 1990s* (Washington, D.C.: American Psychiatric Press, 1994); K. Heilbrun and L. Peters, "The efficacy and effectiveness of community treatment programmes in preventing crime and violence among those with severe mental illness in the community," in Sheilagh Hodgins, ed., *Violence among the Mentally Ill: Effective Treatments and Management Strategies* (Dordrecht: Kluwer Academic Publishers, 1999), pp. 341–58.

24. *Kendra's Law: Final Report on the Status of Assisted Outpatient Treatment* (New York State Office of Mental Health, March 2005).

25. G. Zanni and L. deVeau, "Inpatient stays before and after outpatient commitment," *Hospital and Community Psychiatry* 37 (1986): 941–42.

26. G. A. Fernandez and S. Nygard, "Impact of involuntary outpatient commitment on the revolving-door syndrome in North Carolina," *Hospital and Community Psychiatry* 41 (1990): 1001–4.

27. M. R. Munetz, T. Grande, J. Kleist, et al., "The effectiveness of outpatient civil commitment," *Psychiatric Services* 47 (1996): 1251–53.

28. B. M. Rohland, *The Role of Outpatient Commitment in the Management of Persons with Schizophrenia* (Iowa Consortium for Mental Health, Services, Training, and Research, May 1998).

29. M. S. Swartz, J. W. Swanson, H. R. Wagner, et al., "Can involuntary outpatient commitment reduce hospital recidivism?: Findings from a randomized trial with severely mentally ill individuals," *American Journal of Psychiatry* 156 (1999): 1968–75.

30. See note 24 above.

31. V. A. Hiday, M. S. Swartz, J. W. Swanson, et al., "Impact of outpatient commitment on victimization of people with severe mental illness," *American Journal of Psychiatry* 159 (2002): 1403–11.

32. J. W. Swanson, R. Borum, M. S. Swartz, et al., "Can involuntary outpatient commitment reduce arrests among persons with severe mental illness?" *Criminal Justice and Behavior* 28 (2001): 156–89.

33. See note 24 above.

34. J. W. Swanson, M. S. Swartz, R. Borum, et al., "Involuntary out-patient commitment and reduction of violent behaviour in persons with severe mental illness," *British Journal of Psychiatry* 176 (2000): 324–31.

35. See note 24 above.

36. B. Bursten, "Posthospital mandatory outpatient treatment," *American Journal of Psychiatry* 143 (1986): 1255–58.

37. See note 24 above.

38. H. I. Schwartz, W. Vingiano, and C. Bezirganian Perez, "Autonomy and the right to refuse treatment: Patients' attitudes after involuntary medication," *Hospital and Community Psychiatry* 39 (1988): 1049–54; N. H. S. Adams and R. J. Hafner, "Attitudes of psychiatric patients and their relatives to involuntary treatment," *Australian and New Zealand Journal of Psychiatry* 25 (1991): 231–37; H. Variainen, O. Vuorio, P. Halonen, et al., "The patients' opinions about curative factors in involuntary treatment," *Acta Psychiatrica Scandinavica* 91 (1995): 163–66; A. Lucksted and R. D. Coursey, "Consumer perceptions of pressure and force in psychiatric treatments," *Psychiatric Services* 46 (1995): 146–52; W. M. Greenberg, L. Moore-Duncan, and R. Herron, "Patients' attitudes toward having been forcibly medicated," *Bulletin of the American Academy of Psychiatry and the Law* 24 (1996): 513–24.

39. See note 24 above.

40. L. O. Gostin, "Controlling the resurgent tuberculosis epidemic," *Law and Medicine* 269 (1993): 255–61; M. R. Gasner, K. L. Maw, G. E. Feldman, et al., "The use of legal action in New York City to ensure treatment of tuberculosis," *New England Journal of Medicine* 340 (1999): 359–66.

41. G. A. Ellard, P. J. Jenner, and P. A. Downs, "An evaluation of the potential use of isoniazid, acetylisoniazid, and isonicortinic acid for monitoring the self-administration of drugs," *British Journal of Clinical Pharmacology* 10 (1980): 369–81; P. M. Edelbrook, F. G. Zitman, J. N. Schreinder, et al., "Amitriptyline metabolism in relation to antidepressant effect," *Clinical Pharmacology and Therapeutics* 35 (1984): 467–73.

CHAPTER 12: CODA: DEATH BY THE ROADSIDE

1. Unless otherwise noted, all quotations are taken from the trial transcript or the transcript of the appeal, accessed in the South Carolina Supreme Court library.

2. D. Suchetka, "Suspect testifies she shot brother out of fear," *Charlotte Observer*, May 24, 1989; "I love you, woman said, then killed brother," *Rock Hill Herald*, May 24, 1989.

3. A. D. Helms, "Psychotics turned out, doctor says," *Charlotte Observer*, April 27, 1989; transcript of appeal, Lothell Tate versus the State, October 16, 1990; letter from Eugene Maloney to E. Fuller Torrey, August 2006.

4. D. Suchetka and B. Martin, "A diseased mind, a desperate act, relatives sought to end nightmare with gunfire," *Charlotte Observer*, February 26, 1989; K. Garloch, "Rights of mentally ill making helping hard," ibid., March 20, 1989; letter from E. Fuller Torrey to Lothell Tate, March 2, 1989.

5. C. Acker and M. J. Fine, "Families under siege: A mental health crisis," *Philadelphia Inquirer*, September 10, 1989.

6. A. Bumgarner, "Shooting death investigated," *G-K-K News*, July 3, 1986; letter from Virginia M. Gliddon to Governor James R. Thompson, September 3, 1986.

7. Acker and Fine, "Families under siege."

8. D. Suchetka, "Woman gets life for murdering schizophrenic brother," *Charlotte Observer*, May 25, 1989.

9. M. Wynn, "10-year prison term cut to one for woman who hid son's murder," *Charlotte Observer*, August 16, 1989; interview with Pauline Wilkerson, July 14, 2005.

10. M. P. Jackson and P. Zerwick, "Breakdown: A crisis in mental-health care," *Winston-Salem Journal*, December 4, 2005.

11. L. Bonner, "Scarcity of mental-health care traps patients in vicious cycle," *Raleigh News and Observer*, March 9, 2007.

12. M. P. Jackson, "Nowhere to go: State hospital moving patients into area's homeless shelters," *Winston-Salem Journal*, February 5, 2006.

13. J. Burgess, "Nurse sees jail as 'dumping ground' for many of the mentally ill," *Hendersonville Times News*, January 4, 2006.

14. M. Brumley, "Involuntary commitments strain police manpower," *Asheboro Courier-Tribune*, January 9, 2006; Jackson and Zerwick, "Breakdown."

15. E. J. S. Townsend, "Mixed populations in assisted living concerns advocates," *Greensboro News-Record*, August 20, 2006; M. P. Jackson and P. Zerwick, "Risky: Patients sent to family-care homes," *Winston-Salem Journal*, December 4, 2005.

16. Accounts taken from Preventable Tragedies database, www.treatmentadvocacy center.org.

17. L. Setegn, "Man sentenced in son's death," *Richmond Times-Dispatch*, April 20, 2004.
18. D. Cahn, "Dad devastated by triple slaying: Son held in deaths of mom, sister, nephew," *Middletown Times Herald-Record*, September 17, 2004.
19. B. Martin, "Man has sympathy for slaying victim, suspects—all kin," *Charlotte Observer*, December 25, 1988.

APPENDIX A

1. S. E. Estroff, C. Zimmer, W. S. Lachicotte, et al., "The influence of social networks and social support on violence by persons with serious mental illness," *Hospital and Community Psychiatry* 45 (1994): 669–78; S. E. Estroff and C. Zimmer, "Social networks, social support, and violence among persons with severe, persistent mental illness," in J. Monahan and H. Steadman, *Violence and Mental Disorder: Developments in Risk Assessment* (Chicago: University of Chicago Press, 1994); J. Swanson, S. Estroff, M. Swartz, et al., "Violence and severe mental disorder in clinical and community populations: The effects of psychotic symptoms, comorbidity, and lack of treatment," *Psychiatry* 60 (1997): 1–22.
2. B. G. Link, H. Andrews, and P. T. Cullen, "The violent and illegal behavior of mental patients reconsidered," *American Sociological Review* 57 (1992): 275–92; B. G. Link and A. Stueve, "Psychotic symptoms and the violent/illegal behavior of mental patients compared to community controls," in Monahan and Steadman, *Violence and Mental Disorder*, pp. 137–59.
3. J. W. Swanson, C. E. Holzer, V. K. Ganju, et al., "Violence and psychiatric disorder in the community: Evidence from the Epidemiologic Catchment Area Surveys," *Hospital and Community Psychiatry* 41 (1990): 761–70; J. W. Swanson, "Mental disorder, substance abuse, and community violence: An epidemiological approach," in Monahan and Steadman, *Violence and Mental Disorder*, pp. 101–36.
4. H. J. Steadman, E. P. Mulvey, J. Monahan, et al., "Violence by people discharged from acute psychiatric inpatient facilities and by others in the same neighborhoods," *Archives of General Psychiatry* 55 (1998): 393–401; H. J. Steadman and E. Silver, "Immediate precursors of violence among persons with mental illness: A return to a situational perspective," in *Violence among the Mentally Ill* (Boston: Kluwer Academic Publishers, 1999), pp. 35–48.
5. J. W. Swanson, M. S. Swartz, S. M. Essock, et al., "The social-environmental context of violent behavior in persons treated for severe mental illness," *American Journal of Public Health* 92 (2002): 1523–31.
6. J. Monahan, H. J. Steadman, P. C. Robbins, et al., "An actuarial model of violence risk assessment for persons with mental disorders," *Psychiatric Services* 56 (2005): 810–15.
7. J. W. Swanson, M. S. Swartz, R. A. Van Dorn, et al., "A national study of violent behavior in persons with schizophrenia," *Archives of General Psychiary* 63 (2006): 490–99.
8. J. W. Swanson, R. A. Van Dorn, J. Monahan, et al., "Violence and leveraged community treatment for persons with mental disorders," *American Journal of Psychiatry* 163 (2006): 1404–11.

9. E. B. Elbogen, R. A. Van Dorn, J. W. Swanson, et al. "Treatment engagement and violence risk in mental disorders," *British Journal of Psychiatry* 189 (2006): 354–60.

APPENDIX B

1. H. Gillies, "Homicide in the west of Scotland," *British Journal of Psychiatry* 128 (1976): 105–27.
2. H. Hafner and W. Boker, *Crimes of Violence by Mentally Abnormal Offenders: A Psychiatric and Epidemiological Study in the Federal German Republic* (Cambridge: Cambridge University Press, 1982).
3. P. Gottlieb, G. Gabrielsen, and P. Kramp, "Psychotic homicides in Copenhagen from 1959 to 1983," *Acta Psychiatrica Scandinavica* 76 (1987): 285–92.
4. M. Wong and K. Singer, "Abnormal homicide in Hong Kong," *British Journal of Psychiatry* 123 (1973): 295–98.
5. C. Evans and R. R. Malesu, "Homicide in Barbados: An 18-year review," *Journal of Forensic Psychiatry* 12 (2001): 182–93.
6. P. J. Taylor and J. Gunn, "Violence and psychosis: I. Risk of violence among psychotic men," *British Medical Journal* 288 (1984): 1945–49.
7. G. Coté and S. Hodgins, "The prevalence of major mental disorders among homicide offenders," *International Journal of Law and Psychiatry* 15 (1992): 89–99.
8. A. I. F. Simpson, B. McKenna, A. Moskowitz, et al., "Homicide and mental illness in New Zealand," 185 (2004): 394–98.
9. H. Schanda, G. Knecht, D. Schreinzer, et al., "Homicide and major mental disorders: A 25-year study," *Acta Psychiatrica Scandinavica* 110 (2004): 98–107; H. Schanda, personal communication, October 28, 2004.
10. M. Eronen, P. Hakola, and J. Tiihonen, "Mental disorders and homicidal behavior in Finland," *Archives of General Psychiatry* 53 (1996): 497–501; M. Eronen, J. Tiihonen, and P. Hakola, "Schizophrenia and homicidal behavior," *Schizophrenia Bulletin* 22 (1996): 83–89.
11. S. Fazel and M. Grann, "Psychiatric morbidity among homicide offenders: A Swedish population study," *American Journal of Psychiatry* 161 (2004): 2129–31.
12. M. Erb, S. Hodgins, R. Freese, et al., "Homicide and schizophrenia: Maybe treatment does have a preventive effect," *Criminal Behaviour and Mental Health* 11 (2001): 6–26.
13. C. Wallace, P. Mullen, P. Burgess, et al., "Serious criminal offending and mental disorder," *British Journal of Psychiatry* 172 (1998): 477–84.
14. J. Shaw, L. Appleby, and T. Amos, "Mental disorder and clinical care in people convicted of homicide: National clinical survey," *British Medical Journal* 318 (1999): 1240–44; Shaw, I. M. Hunt, S. A. Flynn, et al., "Rates of mental disorder in people convicted of homicide," *British Journal of Psychiatry* 188 (2005): 143–47; J. Meehan, S. Flynn, I. M. Hunt, et al., "Perpetrators of homicide with schizophrenia: A national clinical survey in England and Wales," *Psychiatric Services* 57 (2006): 1648–51.
15. L. Appleby and J. Shaw, "Five-year report of the national confidential inquiry into suicide and homicide by people with mental illness," available at www.medicine

.manchester.ac.uk/suicideprevention/nci/Useful/avoidable_deaths_full_report.pdf, accessed August 2, 2007.

16. K. G. W. W. Koh, K. P. Gwee, and Y. H. Chan, "Psychiatric aspects of homicide in Singapore: A five-year review," *Singapore Medicine* 47 (2006): 297–304.

17. O. B. Nielssen, B. D. Westmore, M. M. B. Large, et al., "Homicide during psychotic illness in New South Wales between 1993 and 2002," *Medical Journal of Australia* 186 (2007): 301–4.

Index

Page numbers in *italics* refer to figures and tables.

251